1. What is the estimated contraceptive failure rate of the pill? Of condoms?

2. What is a sign that a fetus is in serious trouble?

3. If you have swollen, bleeding gums, is that normal?

4. There are four signs of true versus false labor. Can you name one?

5. Can you breast-feed if you have had a breast reduction operation? Breast augmentation?

6. How many diapers a day should a breast-fed infant wet?

ISN'T IT IMPORTANT THAT YOU HAVE THE FACTS? YOUR LIFE AND YOUR HEALTH MAY DEPEND ON IT.

Answers:

1. *6%; 16%*
2. *Decreased fetal movement for 12 hours after week 28*
3. *Yes*
4. *In false labor, contractions are irregular and do not get closer, stop with movement, are felt in the abdomen, and do not get stronger. True labor contractions are regular and get closer together, are continuous in spite of movement, are usually felt in the back first, and increase steadily in strength.*
5. *Probably yes. Yes.*
6. *Six*

The American Medical Women's Association

Guide to Pregnancy and Childbirth

Medical Co-editors
**Roselyn Payne Epps, M.D., M.P.H., M.A., F.A.A.P.
Susan Cobb Stewart, M.D., F.A.C.P.**

A Dell Book

Published by
Dell Publishing
a division of
Bantam Doubleday Dell Publishing Group, Inc.
1540 Broadway
New York, New York 10036

This material was originally published along with other material
in THE WOMEN'S COMPLETE HEALTHBOOK published by
Delacorte Press.

Illustrations by Wendy Frost

ISBN: 0-440-22246-X

Reprinted by arrangement with Delacorte Press

Printed in the United States of America

Published simultaneously in Canada

July 1996

10 9 8 7 6 5 4 3 2 1

OPM

The AMWA Guide to Pregnancy and Childbirth

Roselyn Payne Epps, M.D., M.P.H., M.A.,
and Susan Cobb Stewart, M.D.

The time from conception to childbirth is one of great joy, excitement, and anticipation for women. For many, however, it can also be a challenging experience fraught with confusing and strenuous physical changes. To monitor and understand the bodily changes that occur during pregnancy, women need a definitive source for accurate, dependable, and up-to-date information. *The AMWA Guide to Pregnancy and Childbirth* presents essential information developed by the American Medical Women's Association (AMWA), the most prestigious association of women physicians in the world. The authors are all women physicians with an in-depth understanding of the female reproductive system.

AMWA believes that women must avoid a disease-oriented approach to women's health and focus on maintaining optimal health on a daily and long-term basis. The more a woman knows about her body and its functions, the better equipped she will be to safeguard good health through preventive strategies such as eating properly and exercising regularly. The content of *The AMWA Guide to Pregnancy and Childbirth* is divided ito three major sections:

Part I, The Reproductive System, provides thorough descriptions of both female and male reproductive systems, from early development to mature function. It recommends preventive strategies for maintaining good reproductive health, and covers conditions and illnesses of the female system and how to approach them.

Part II, Pregnancy and Childbirth, begins with a prepregnancy health evaluation that shows women how to prepare their bodies for the healthiest possible pregnancy. It subsequently discusses all phases of fetal development, carefully explaining what women experience during these months. This section also explores the processes of labor and delivery as well as postpregnancy, and helps inform women of their options should depression set in.

Part III, Breast-feeding, introduces all of the successful breast-feeding techniques. It explains why breast-feeding is beneficial to both mother and child, and supplies information on where to get further assistance should complications rise.

The AMWA Guide to Pregnancy and Childbirth provides authoritative information that all women need in today's changing environment. It illuminates health concerns unique to women of the 1990s and offers sound medical advice. Supported by the expertise and experience of the American Medical Women's Association, *The AMWA Guide to Pregnancy and Childbirth* offers a sensitive and sensible approach to helping women achieve a healthy, happy pregnancy, childbirth, and postpregnancy recovery.

CONTENTS

PART III
BREAST-FEEDING
Ruth A. Lawrence, M.D., F.A.A.P.

The American Medical Women's Association

Guide to Pregnancy and Childbirth

PART I
The Reproductive System

Katherine A. O'Hanlan, M.D.,
F.A.C.O.G., F.A.C.S.,
and Jean L. Fourcroy, M.D., PH.D.

The organs that form the reproductive system allow humans to reproduce. Men and women have different reproductive systems that work in unison to create new life. If something goes awry with the components of the female or male reproductive system, it can affect not only the ability to have children but may also cause serious disorders warranting early detection and treatment.

STRUCTURE AND FUNCTION

The reproductive and genital organs of a fetus form during the fourth week of pregnancy. At that time, nerve, blood vessel, and tissue bundles form in patterns that distinguish males from females when they are fully developed. Development of these organs in the fetus ends during the first trimester. (See Fig. 1.1).

Many of the anatomic structures in one sex correspond to those in the other. For instance, The female clitoris and the male penis are derived from the same structures, contain the same number of nerves, and are the site of intense sensitivity during sexual activity.

A child is born with male or female reproductive organs, but these organs remain undeveloped until puberty. Then a spurt of hormones causes rapid growth and development of reproductive organs, changing body structure and function and making a person capable of reproduction.

Females usually mature sexually between the ages of 10 and 14, when the ovaries begin producing the hormone estrogen. This causes the hips to widen, breasts to develop, and body hair to grow. It also triggers menstruation, the monthly cycle of bleeding that is a key part of a woman's fertility. Women continue to produce estrogen and menstruate until about age 50. The amount of estrogen produced by her ovaries slowly decreases until a woman reaches menopause, when her periods stop and she is no longer able to become pregnant naturally.

Males develop sexually a little later than females. At puberty, the hormone testosterone causes an increase in height, muscle development, and the growth of the sex organs, which then produce sperm. Boys may have nocturnal emissions of semen, or wet dreams, at puberty. Around age 50, the production of testosterone in men may decrease. Although lowered levels of testosterone do not seem to affect the ability to have an erection, it may result in a decrease in sexual desire.

The Female Reproductive System

A woman's external genital area is called the vulva. It is made up of the labia minora—the inner lips enclosing the opening to the vagina—and the labia majora—the outer, hair-bearing lips surrounding the opening of the vagina and the urethra, the opening to the bladder. The clitoris is a small bud-shaped organ, located just above the urethra. It is the most sensitive area of the external female genitals. Bartholin's glands are located on either side of the vaginal opening.

The vagina is a muscular tube leading from the external genital organs to the uterus. The opening of the uterus, the cervix, projects into the upper end of the vagina. (See Fig. 1.2). It varies in shape and size

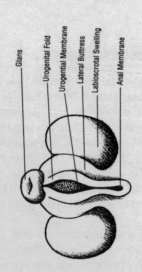

Glans
Urogenital Fold
Urogential Membrane
Lateral Buttress
Labioscrotal Swelling
Anal Membrane

Figure 1.1 Fetal Genitalia
The fetus's external genitalia develop during early pregnancy. Both male and female genitalia arise from the same structure (top), which has begun to form by about 4-7 weeks of gestation. The *glans* gives rise to either the male glans of the penis (bottom left) or the female clitoris (bottom right). The *urogenital membrane* will eventually develop into the urethra, and the *labioscrotal swelling* will form either the male scrotum or the female labia

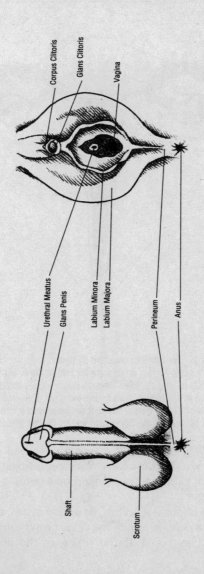

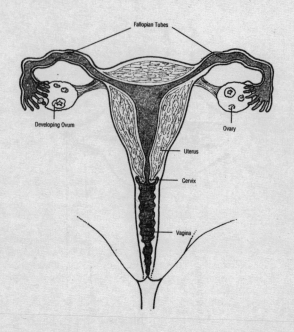

Figure 1.2 Female Reproductive System
A woman's reproductive organs are located in the lower abdomen. Each month, an egg released from an *ovary* moves through a *fallopian tube* to the *uterus*. If an egg is fertilized, it is embedded in the inner wall of the uterus, where it develops into a fetus. The fetus passes through the *cervix* and *vagina* during delivery.

depending on whether a woman has had children. The cervix can be felt by inserting a finger into the vagina. It cannot be penetrated by a penis, a tampon, or a finger.

The uterus is a hollow, muscular organ, about the size of a pear, in which the fetus grows during pregnancy. (See Fig. 1.3) The lining of the uterus, the

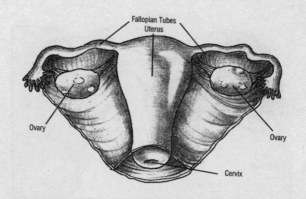

Figure 1.3 The Uterus
The uterus (seen here from the back) is a hollow, muscular organ that varies in size and shape. In women who have not had children, it usually measures about two and a half to a little over three inches long. In women who have had children, it ranges from about three and a half to four inches long.

endometrium, changes in thickness depending on a woman's menstrual cycle. The fallopian tubes extend from either side of the upper end of the uterus. They are about 4 inches in length and reach outward toward the ovaries. (See Fig. 1.4) The ovaries are the female sex organs that produce eggs and female hormones.

A woman is born with 2 million undeveloped eggs in her ovaries—more than enough to last during her reproductive life. Each month, an egg matures in the ovaries and is released into the fallopian tubes. This process is called ovulation. If a man and a woman have sex at that time and the man's sperm unites with the woman's egg, fertilization occurs. The fertilized egg then moves into the woman's uterus

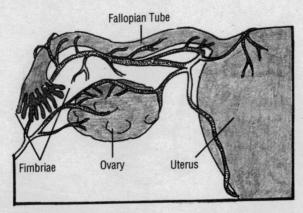

Figure 1.4 The Fallopian Tubes
The fallopian tubes extend outward from either side of the uterus. At the end of each tube, fingerlike projections called *fimbriae* are situated close to the surface of the ovary. During ovulation, the egg released by one of the ovaries enters the tube through the fimbriae.

where it becomes attached to the endometrium and begins to grow into a fetus. (See Fig. 1.5) If the egg is not fertilized, it dissolves in her body. The endometrium, which thickens before ovulation to prepare for the fertilized egg, begins to break down and menstruation, or bleeding occurs. The hormones estrogen and progesterone, produced in the ovaries, regulate the menstrual cycle (see "Hormones of the Reproductive System").

Estrogen is secreted by the ovaries throughout a woman's reproductive years, affecting all the cells of the body. Special estrogen receptors are located in the breasts, the lining of the uterus, the cervix, and the upper vagina. Cells with estrogen receptors grow when estrogen is in the blood, whether it is secreted from the ovaries or taken in pill form. The lining of the

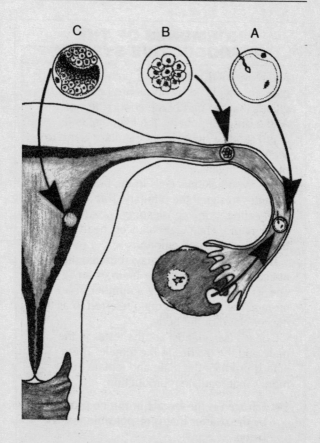

Figure 1.5 Fertilization
The process of fertilization begins with the release of an egg from one of the ovaries. Normally, penetration of an egg by a sperm occurs in the far end of a fallopian tube (A) anywhere from 12 to 24 hours after ovulation. By the time the fertilized egg has reached the near end of the tube (B), it has already begun to divide. Implantation in the wall of the uterus (C) usually occurs 3-4 days after ovulation.

HORMONES OF THE REPRODUCTIVE SYSTEM

The reproductive systems of both women and men are regulated by hormones produced by glands that are part of the endocrine system. At the onset of puberty, the hypothalamus gland sends a signal to the pituitary gland to secrete hormones that cause the development of sexual organs.

The hypothalamus cells in the brain secrete peptides to signal the pituitary. This area regulates eating, drinking, sleeping, waking, body temperature, chemical balances, heart rate, hormones, sex, and emotions.

The pituitary, a small, gray, rounded gland attached to the base of the brain, is an endocrine gland secreting a number of hormones. The pituitary is often referred to as the master gland of the body.

Gonads (sex glands) are the testes in the male and the ovaries in the female. These glands produce the male and female hormones that regulate reproduction:

- Estrogen is the female hormone produced by the ovaries that is responsible for ovulation.
- Progesterone is a female hormone produced by the ovaries after ovulation. It triggers the menstrual period. It prepares the uterine lining for the fertilized egg.

■ Testosterone is the gonadal steroid secreted by the male. After puberty, the normal male secretes testosterone daily. It is responsible for the growth of the prostate and the penis during puberty.

ANABOLIC STEROIDS

Androgens are male sex hormones, one of which is testosterone. Anabolic steroids are synthetic androgens that have been designed to enhance the growth-promoting effects of androgens. Anabolic steriods are occasionally used, under a doctor's supervision, to treat skeletal and growth disorders and certain types of anemia. Steroids are also used illegally, mainly by athletes who want to quickly build muscle tissue. They have many potentially serious side effects: reduced sperm production, decreased size of the testes, and reduced natural sex hormone production, resulting in a diminished sex drive. Steroids can also lead to liver damage and cardiovascular disease and, if taken in early puberty, result in short stature.

uterus has the greatest number of receptors, and it thickens on a monthly basis. Each month, when estrogen levels decline, the lining is broken down and results in a menstrual period.

Progesterone is a hormone secreted by the ovaries after ovulation. It causes the uterine lining cells to stop growing and to simply prepare to nourish an egg should it be fertilized and become implanted in the uterus. At menopause, when ovulation ceases, no more progesterone can be made by the ovaries.

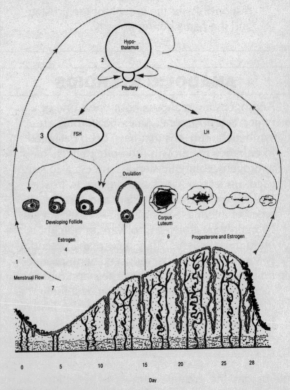

Figure 1.6 The Menstrual Cycle
During the menstrual cycle, an egg is produced, released into a fallopian tube, and eventually, the uterine lining is shed if fertilization does not occur. The average menstrual cycle typically lasts 28 days, but it may vary from 23 to 35 days.

The menstrual cycle is an average of 28 days, although some women have longer or shorter cycles. Ovulation occurs at around day 14 of the cycle (counting from the first day of the previous menstrual period), and it is at this time that a woman can become pregnant. Once released, the egg remains fertile for up to 48 hours. (See Figure 1.6)

1. The cycle begins on day 1 of menstruation, when the lining of the uterus (the *endometrium*) is shed as menstrual blood. Menstruation occurs in response to a decline in the hormones estrogen and progesterone, which occurs when an egg is not fertilized.

2. The decrease in estrogen and progesterone causes the *hypothalamus* to send a message to the *pituitary*.

3. The pituitary in turn releases *follicle-stimulating hormone* (FSH). Follicles are the structures inside the ovaries that produce eggs for fertilization. Each month, one follicle will produce the egg for that cycle.

4. FSH continues to be produced during days 1-13 of the menstrual cycle. Under its influence, the developing follicle begins to produce estrogen. This hormone stimulates the endometrium to grow and thicken in preparation for a fertilized egg. At this time, the mucus normally produced by the cervix becomes thin, clear, and watery.

5. As the developing follicle continues to produce estrogen, the hormone triggers the pituitary to release *luteinizing hormone* (LH). LH stimulates the follicle to release an egg into a fallopian tube. This event, called *ovulation*, typically occurs on day 14 of the cycle.

6. After releasing the egg, the follicle begins to change into a structure known as the *corpus luteum*. This structure then begins to produce the hormone progesterone, which causes the lining of the uterus to continue to thicken in preparation for a fertilized egg.

7. If the egg is not fertilized, a sharp drop occurs in the production of estrogen and progesterone. This triggers the shedding of the endometrium, which marks the start of another menstrual cycle.

The Male Reproductive System

Like that of females, the reproductive system of males is regulated by hormones, which have an effect through birth, puberty, maturity, and aging (see "Hormones of the Reproductive System"). The male genital organs (testes) produce sperm cells and transport them through a series of ducts to the female reproductive system. (See Fig. 1.7)

Each day a male produces about 50 million sperm, the smallest living cells of the body. When a man ejaculates during sexual intercourse, he releases millions of sperm, but only one joins with a woman's egg to fertilize it. Sperm cells can live up to 5 days inside a woman. If a sperm cell joins with a woman's egg released at ovulation, fertilization occurs and a woman becomes pregnant.

The penis, a rod-shaped organ, also transports urine (see Fig. 1.8). Within the penis is the urethra, which carries the urine from the bladder. The penis also holds many blood vessels, which become engorged with blood during sexual excitement, causing an erection (tumescence).

The testes are two egg-shaped organs contained in a pouch of skin called the scrotum that hangs behind the penis. In each of the testicles there is a tightly packed mass of tubes surrounded by a protective capsule. Leydig cells in the testes produce the hormone testosterone, and the tubes in the testes produce sperm. The production of sperm requires a temperature that is lower than the body's internal temperature. Spermatic cords suspend the testicles within the scrotum and help to maintain the correct temperature for sperm production. When the outside temperature is low, the cords draw the testicles upward, nearer to the warm body.

The epididymis is a cordlike structure beside and behind the testes that transports sperm cells from the testicles to the seminal vesicles. Lying behind the bladder, the seminal vesicles store sperm. The sperm are mingled in a fluid that forms part of the semen that is released during ejaculation.

The vas deferens is a thick muscular tube, which is about 1/4 inch in diameter and about 18 inches long. It assists in the transportation and propulsion of sperm and fluid from the testicle in ejaculation. Vasectomy is a method of male sterilization by blocking or cutting the vas deferens.

The prostate is a walnut-shaped gland located below the bladder, surrounding the urethra. Its main function is to produce a fluid that nourishes sperm and helps transport sperm through the urethra during ejaculation.

Cowper's glands, also known as bulbourethral glands, are two teardrop-shaped structures each the size of a pea. They are situated on either side of the urethra and provide mucus and chemicals during sexual excitement. The mucus washes the urethra in preparation for ejaculation and serves as a lubricant.

Semen is the fluid that is ejaculated during the male sexual act. An ejaculation may contain as many as 120,000,000 sperm (see Fig. 1.9). Semen is milky white fluid containing not only sperm but also secretions from the seminal vesicles, prostate gland, and bulbourethral glands. These fluids combine to create the best possible conditions for the survival and function of the sperm. The mucus furnishes lubrication, but initially makes the sperm somewhat immobile. Within about a half hour after ejaculation, however, the fluid dissolves the mucus and the sperm become highly mobile.

Erection of the penis is provoked by sexual stim- ulation. Impulses are transmitted from the brain down the spinal cord to the penis by parasympathetic nerves. The messages signal the corpora cavernosa,

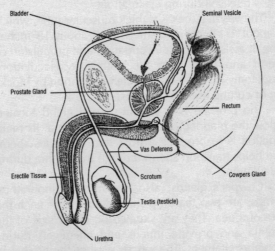

Figure 1.7 The Male Reproductive System
Sperm cells are produced in the *testes*, two roundish organs locat- ed within the *scrotum*. To develop normally, sperm cells need a temperature that is slightly lower (about 95°F) than normal body temperature. The scrotum's location outside the warmer body cavi- ty provides the right conditions for sperm production. After being stored in the *epididymis*, a structure lying next to the testes, sperm cells move through the *vas deferens* and enter the *urethra*. There they are bathed in secretions from the *prostate gland* and the *semi- nal vesicles*, from which semen is formed. With sexual stimulation, secretions from the *bulbourethral glands* help to lubricate the inside of the urethra, and the penis becomes erect. During ejacula- tion, the sperm-containing semen passes through the urethra to the outside of the body. Shown here is a penis with the *foreskin*, a sheath of tissue covering the head (*glans*) of the penis, intact; in many males, the foreskin is removed shortly after birth.

two rod-shaped bundles of muscle in the penis on either side, to relax and fill with blood. As they fill, the corpora cavernosa expand and press against the veins that would normally drain blood from the penis. The penis becomes firm and erect, allowing penetration into the female vagina during sexual intercourse.

Sensations on the skin of the penis that occur during intercourse stimulate the organ's numerous nerve endings. These impulses are carried back to the

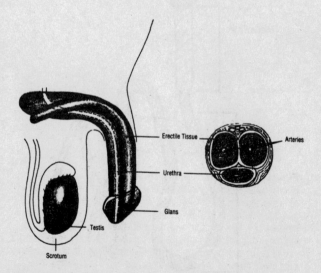

Figure 1.8   Internal Anatomy of the Penis
The shaft of the penis (left) consists of spongy erectile tissue (top right), through which two large arteries and the urethra run length-wise (bottom right). During sexual arousal, blood flow through these arteries increases, and the small veins that normally drain the tissue are temporarily pressed shut. Blood cannot drain, and the penis becomes enlarged and rigid.

brain. The sexual stimulation gradually builds in intensity until it causes a reflex action. Impulses travel down the nerves, passing through the genital organs, and trigger ejaculation, the rhythmic contractions of the smooth muscle of the testicles which

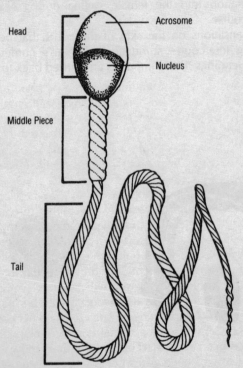

Figure 1.9 Sperm

The head, or *nucleus*, of a sperm cell contains 23 chromosomes. At the tip is the *acrosome*, which contains enzymes that break down barriers surrounding the female ovum. The *middle piece* consists of structures that power cell movement. The rapid movements of the *tail* propel the sperm cell through the female reproductive tract.

expel their contents, the semen, into the urethra. The bulbourethral glands discharge additional amounts of mucus at this time. The act of ejaculation, and the feelings of intense pleasure associated with it, are the male orgasm or climax.

KEEPING THE SYSTEM HEALTHY

Understanding and monitoring your own reproductive system is key to keeping it healthy. Health maintenance involves routine self-examinations, regular checkups, prevention of problems, and being alert to signs of problems so they can be treated early. A number of practitioners treat the reproductive system (see "Health Care Practitioners").

The reproductive systems of both women and men are vulnerable to sexually transmitted diseases (STDs), such as syphilis, gonorrhea, herpes, chlamydia, human papillomavirus (HPV), and AIDS. To protect against STDs, you should limit your sexual partners and always use a condom during sexual intercourse. A woman having sex with another woman should be careful not to have contact with her partner's genital fluids or with any open sores on her partner's body. (The use of a dental dam or cellophane wrap has been advocated but has not been shown to be as clearly of value as the condom is for heterosexuals.) In men, certain STDs can appear as an inflammation of the urethra or a discharge, but also can occur without symptoms. In women, there can be no symptoms. Both women and men should be alert to the early signs of STDs, get treatment immediately, and avoid spreading the disease to others.

SEXUALLY TRANSMITTED DISEASES

Diseases that are sexually transmitted (STDs) can affect both women and men. Often there are no symptoms; when they occur, immediate treatment should be obtained. Both sexual partners must be treated to avoid spreading the disease.

To protect against STDs, women and men should limit their sexual partners. Mutually monogamous relationships and using a condom each time they have sex are the best protection. Spermicides can provide additional protection from STDs. Some of the more common STDs include the following:

- *Chlamydia* is a bacterial infection that can cause urethritis (inflammation of the urethra causing pain, burning, and discharge) in men and pelvic inflammatory disease in women, which can lead to infertility. It is treated with antibiotics.

- *Gonorrhea* is a bacterial infection that can cause urethritis in men and pelvic inflammatory disease in women. It is treated with antibiotics.

- *Herpes* is a viral infection that causes painful blisters on the lips or the genitals. When they are present, the virus can be spread to others. There is no cure but symptoms can be treated.

- *Human papillomavirus* is a viral infection that can cause warts on the external and internal genital area. In women, it can cause abnormal Pap test results and lead to cancer of the cervix. The warts can be removed but there is no real cure for the virus.

- *Syphilis* is an infection whose first sign is a sore on the genitals that may go away, although the infection does not; it can lead to long-term disability. Syphilis is treated with antibiotics.

- *Trichomonas* is an infection caused by overgrowth of an organism in the vagina, causing a frothy discharge and itching. It is treated with a drug called metronidazole.

For Women

Every woman's genitals are shaped individually, with different sizes for inner lips, outer lips, and clitoris. Women of all ages should be familiar with the appearance of their genitals and be aware of what is normal for them. In this way, changes that may be the only signs of certain infections or precancerous conditions can be detected early. Early diagnosis means conditions can be diagnosed and treated before they have advanced to later stages. Small sores, ulcers, raw areas, or pigmented areas can be the first and earliest signs of cancer of the vulva. Use a mirror to inspect your vulva monthly to look for these signs.

Women should protect themselves from unwanted pregnancy by using some method of birth control. Ideally, the birth control method should also protect against infections; a barrier method, such as a condom, is ideal. Of course not all methods are perfect, and failures of contraception do occur. Early diagnosis of a missed period allows your maximum choice in expression of your reproductive desires. If you have had sex without birth control or your birth control has failed, ask your doctor about postcoital, or emergency, contraception.

You should have a pelvic examination and a Pap test annually to detect changes in the cervix that could be early signs of cancer (see "The Pap Test"). (See Fig. 1.10A-B). Depending on your situation, your doctor may suggest you have this done more or less often. Any unusual bleeding, pain, or discharge should be brought to the attention of a doctor.

The Pap Test

The Pap test was named after Dr. George Papanicolaou, the physician who developed it. A Pap test can detect changes in the cells on the cervix that could be early signs of cancer. For the test, a women lies on an examining table with her feet in stirrups. An instrument called a speculum is inserted into her vagina to hold it open. With a small brush or scraper, a sample of cells is removed from the cervix and placed on a glass slide so it can be studied under a microscope.

If menstruation starts and is heavy at the time of an appointment, the appointment should be rescheduled. Also, a woman should not douche before the test.

Test results are reported in categories according to the Bethesda system. A negative result means that there are no abnormal cells present in the sample of cells. A positive result means that some abnormal cells are present and may require further testing. As with any test, however, the results depend on the quality of the lab work and the person evaluating the cells.

The Pap test has greatly reduced the number of deaths from cancer of the cervix, and is used to prevent cervical cancer. The test should be performed annually, with a pelvic exam, for women who have been sexually active or who have reached the age of 18. If results are normal for three consecutive years, the woman is in a monogamous relationship or is celibate, and has no risk factors such as infection with human papillomavirus or smoking, she may then have a Pap test every three years. Many physicians feel that a yearly Pap test will better detect abnormal cells that can develop into cancer.

For Men

Recognition and treatment of problems that can arise in the reproductive system as a man ages are essential for a healthy life. Men should have regular checkups to watch for early signs of problems. For example, signs of prostate enlargement include changes or problems with urination such as more frequent urination, a feeling of a need to urinate, and a weak stream of urine. The checkup should include a thorough history and a physical examination. The history should include a family history as well as an occupational and medical history, past genitourinary surgery, or trauma to the reproductive organs. Men should ask their doctors questions regarding any illnesses, changes in sex drive, or drugs that may interfere with reproductive health.

Prostate gland enlargement does not increase the risk of prostate cancer, but cancer could be present at the same time or develop later. Many older men have

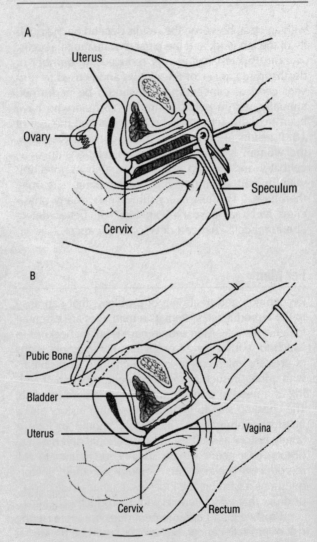

some symptoms of prostate enlargement. All men over age 50 should have digital rectal examinations once a year to detect prostate cancer. The digital rectal exam involves the insertion of a finger into the rectum to feel the prostate. This important part of total health care can detect enlargement, abnormal texture, or hard areas of the prostate that could be signs of cancer.

Men of all ages should perform testicular self-examination monthly to detect problems that could be a sign of cancer of the testes. It only takes a few minutes and can be done easily and painlessly, preferably after a warm bath or shower or in a warm room when the scrotum is relaxed. To perform the exam, roll each testicle between the thumbs and fore-fingers of both hands. Any hard lumps or nodules should be brought to the attention of a physician.

SYMPTOMS

Any signs or symptoms of problems in the reproductive system warrant medical attention. In women,

Figure 1.10   Tests
A woman should have a gynecologic exam, including a Pap smear, at least once a year or more if her doctor advises it. The Pap test (A) is performed by inserting an instrument called a *speculum* into the vagina to hold the walls of the vagina apart. A small spatula or brush is then used to collect a sample of cells from the cervix. The cell sample is then smeared onto a glass slide, which is examined under a microscope. A biannual pelvic exam (B) is recommended for every woman on a regular basis. For this exam, the doctor feels the shape, size, and position of the internal reproductive organs by inserting two fingers into the vagina and pressing down on the abdomen with the other hand. Many doctors also perform a rectal exam afterward.

problems that can signal a disorder include abnormal bleeding or discharge, pain, or a change in the appearance of the genital organs. In men, changes in their urination or pain can signal prostate enlargement or cancer. In both women and men, any unusual lump or growth that can be felt or seen should receive medical attention.

In Women

In young women, any irregular bleeding may be linked to problems with the hormones secreted by the ovaries. In older women, changes in their menstrual periods could signal menopause. Some women may have irregular, unpredictable, and sometimes heavy bleeding during menopause. They have a slightly higher chance of developing precancerous or cancerous changes of the endometrium and should be monitored by a physician. An endometrial biopsy can determine whether precancerous changes are taking place. In this technique, a sample of the tissue lining the uterus is obtained and studied. After menopause, when a woman has stopped having menstrual periods for 12 months, any bleeding should be evaluated.

It is normal for women to have a clear vaginal discharge. This discharge cleans the vagina, maintains its normal state, and keeps it free of organisms. A discharge that is white or yellow, thick or frothy, or has an odor could be a sign of an infection. Itching also may occur. These symptoms could signal a major or minor problem; have them checked so the cause can be identified and treated.

Pain in the pelvic area can occur for many reasons, although it is usually due to either a cramping of the uterus or conditions affecting the ovaries. Pain in the pelvic region also can be related to any of the anatomic structures in this area, including the ureters, bladder, and rectum. If the pain is sudden, severe, and long lasting, or interferes with daily activities, consult your physician.

A pain in your right or left side can be a sign of ovulation. This pain, called *mittelschmerz* (literally, middle pain), is caused by the release of the egg. It may be accompanied by a clear vaginal discharge and increased sex drive. On rare occasions, there may be slight bleeding.

In Men

Certain symptoms can signal problems with the prostate in men. Many older men have enlarged prostate glands, but this condition does not lead to cancer. Prostate cancer is common in older men, however, so it should be considered when symptoms such as the following are present:

- Hesitant, interrupted, or weak stream of urine
- A sense of urgency, leaking, or dribbling of urine
- More frequent need to urinate, especially at night
- Difficulty starting or holding back urination
- Inability to urinate
- Weak flow of urine
- Painful urination or bloody urine
- Painful ejaculation

■ Pain in the lower back, hips, upper thighs

Any of these symptoms requires further evaluation by a primary care physician or, if necessary, a urologist.

CONDITIONS AND DISORDERS IN WOMEN

The female reproductive system is a fairly complicated mechanism that sustains the monthly cycles that are part of fertility as well as pregnancy and childbirth. Because of the complexity of the reproductive organs and the functions needed to maintain them, some normal conditions as well as disorders may require regular medical attention.

Birth Control

Many methods of birth control, or contraception, are available that have a very high degree of safety and effectiveness (see "Contraceptive Failure Rates"). These methods allow you to choose if and when you wish to have children and to plan your family just as you plan other aspects of your life. Without such methods, up to 85 percent of sexually active women using no contraception would be expected to become pregnant in a year. Some methods, such as condoms and spermicides, also provide protection against STDs and cancer of the cervix. All of them allow you control over your reproduction (see "Women's Choices About Contraception").

CONTRACEPTIVE FAILURE RATES*

Method	Percentage of Average Use†
Contraceptive implants	0.05%
Vasectomy	0.2
Contraceptive injections	0.4
Tubal sterilization	0.5
IUD	4.0
Pill	6.0
Condom (male)‡	16.0
Cervical cap	18.0
Diaphragm	18.0
Periodic abstinence	19.0
Sponge	24.0
Withdrawal	24.0
Condom (female)‡	26.0
Spermicides	30.0
No method (chance)	85.0

*The failure rate is the estimated percentage of all women using the method who will have an unplanned pregnancy in the first year of use.

†Using a method consistently and correctly—the right way, all the time—makes birth control more effective than these rates show.

‡These methods are most effective against sexually transmitted diseases.

Hormonal Methods

Pregnancy can be prevented by using hormones to regulate fertility. The hormone estrogen prevents ovulation, the release of an egg. The hormone progesterone blocks the release of the egg during ovulation, although not as well as estrogen, and creates an environment in the uterine lining that makes pregnancy unlikely. These hormones may be used alone or in combination, depending on the technique.

WOMEN'S CHOICES ABOUT CONTRACEPTION

A woman's choice about which method of birth control to use is largely affected by whether she wishes to have children in the future. Women who do wish to have children choose oral contraceptives most often (49 percent), whereas those who do not plan to have children or who have completed their families choose sterilization (61 percent). About 10 percent of women do not use any form of birth control. These women account for approximately 53 percent of all unintended pregnancies in the United States, half of which end in abortion. Women who are sexually active and not planning to become pregnant should exercise their options of birth control to avoid unintended pregnancy.

Among all women, these are the percentages of women who select specific methods:

Oral contraceptives	27.7%
Tubal sterilization	24.8
Condom	13.1
Periodic abstinence	2.1
IUD	1.8
Spermicides	1.7
Sponge	1

Hormones are used for postcoital, or emergency, contraception, also known as the morning after pill. A doctor or family planning clinic can prescribe the pill, which is usually a combination of birth control pills taken at specific intervals. This technique can be used if a woman has had unprotected intercourse because her method failed or she was sexually assaulted or for any number of reasons. The morning after pill must be administered within hours of intercourse to be effective.

Oral Contraceptives

Birth control pills, or oral contraceptives, are very effective when used properly. There are two types of birth control pills: combination pills, containing the hormones estrogen and progestin, and mini-pills containing only progestin. Progestin is a synthetic version of the natural female hormone progesterone. Women use the combination pills most often; those women who cannot take estrogen use the mini-pill.

To be effective, the pill must be taken regularly. Some pills are taken daily during a 28-day cycle, whereas others are taken for 21 days, with no pills taken for 7 days before the next pack is started. Missing one pill can result in pregnancy. Birth control pills are generally safe for women in good health who do not smoke. There is no reason to have rest periods from oral contraceptives after they are taken for a number of years.

Aside from preventing pregnancy, birth control pills have other benefits. Oral contraceptives protect against cancer of the ovary and the endometrium. The longer a woman takes the pill, the greater the protective effect. Women who take the pill have a lower risk of ovarian cysts, ovarian and endometrial cancer, uterine fibroids, noncancerous breast disease, and ectopic pregnancies. They also tend to have more regular periods with less monthly flow and fewer premenstrual symptoms. The estrogen in oral contraceptives also appears to increase bone density, reducing the risk of bone loss that occurs during menopause.

On the other hand, oral contraceptives have been linked to certain types of cardiovascular disease and cancer of the breast. These effects were observed when higher dose formulations were in use and other factors linked to disease, such as smoking, were not taken into consideration. In general, today's low-dose pills do not seem to pose the same risk. There is, however, an increased risk of thromboembolism (blood clots) in women who smoke and take the pill. Although one study has shown a link between breast cancer and oral contraceptives, others have not been able to confirm that finding.

Oral contraceptives can be used by most healthy women. Do not take birth control pills, however, if any of the following factors apply to you:

- Age over 35 and smoke
- History of vascular disease (including stroke and thromboembolism)
- Uncontrolled high blood pressure, diabetes with vascular disease, high cholesterol
- Active liver disease
- Cancer of the endometrium or breast

Women over age 35 who do not smoke can continue to take a low-dose pill with safety until menopause. Some women may develop bloating, spotting, severe mood swings, or breast tenderness. These problems, or a tendency toward them, require that the woman and her physician work together to find the right formula for her.

Implants
Implants involve a new technique of inserting small plastic tubes containing a progestin or lev-

onorgestrel just under the skin of the arm (see Fig. 1.11). After an injection of local anesthetic to numb the area, the small tubes are imbedded under the skin in the upper arm during an office visit. The hormone is slowly released over a 5-year period. This method of contraception is very effective, but it can cause irregular bleeding and spotting. Other side effects include weight gain, headache, acne, depression, abnormal hair growth, anxiety, and ovarian cysts. The implants need to be surgically removed, and there have been reports that this sometimes can be difficult.

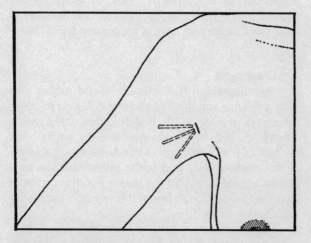

Figure 1.11 Implants
One of the newer methods of birth control is hormonal implants. These small, matchstick-sized tubes are inserted just beneath the surface of the skin, usually on the inner part of a woman's upper arm. The implants contain progestin, a synthetic form of the hormone progesterone, which is slowly released into the bloodstream to prevent pregnancy. Insertion can be done during an office visit, and the implants are effective for up to 5 years.

Injections
The injection technique involves injecting a long-acting type of progesterone into the body every 3 months; the failure rate is low. The side effects with this technique include abdominal discomfort, nervousness, dizziness, decreased sex drive, depression, and acne. Some women have weight gain. This method can disrupt menstrual cycles and cause episodes of bleeding and spotting.

Barrier Methods
Some, but not all, barrier methods provide protection against STDs. They can be used in combination to offer extra protection against pregnancy and STDs.

Diaphragm
The diaphragm is a reusable round rubber disk with a flexible rim that fits inside the vagina to cover the cervix (see Fig. 1.12). It should be coated with a spermicide before it is inserted into the vagina. The success of the diaphragm depends partly on spermicidal cream or jelly and partly on its function as a barrier to block entry of the sperm into the cervix. It must be fitted to the shape of the woman's vagina by a doctor or nurse.

The diaphragm should be inserted 1 hour before intercourse and should be left in place at least 6 hours after having sex. If intercourse is repeated, additional spermicide should be inserted into the vagina. When irritation occurs, it may be due to either the rubber or the spermicide. Changing brands of spermicide may solve this problem.

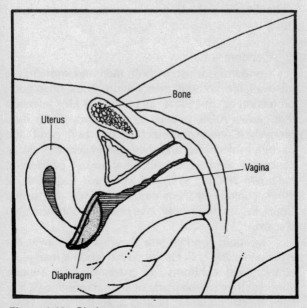

Figure 1.12   Diaphragm
One of the so-called barrier methods of contraception is the diaphragm, a rubber, dome-shaped device that is used with spermicide. It is inserted into the vagina to hold the spermicide in place against the cervix. The flexible rim of the diaphragm helps to hold it in place behind the pubic bone.

Cervical Cap

The cervical cap is similar to the diaphragm, although it is smaller. Fitting snugly over the cervix, it is held in place by suction (see Fig. 1.13). The cervical cap comes in four sizes to fit a woman's cervix. The cervical cap can be difficult to insert, and it doesn't fit all women. It can be left in a longer time than a diaphragm and can be used to contain menstrual fluid.

Condom

Condoms, for use by both men and women, are all available without prescription. They offer good protection against STDs, including the HIV infection that causes AIDS, as well as pregnancy when used properly. Condoms protect against both viral and bacterial infections, and their use lowers the risk of cancer of the cervix. With new sexual partners of unknown risk for STD, use condoms regardless of other contraceptive methods you may be using. Condoms are disposable. Use one time only and then discard.

The *male condom* is a sheath that fits over the erect penis and collects the sperm when a man ejaculates. Most condoms are made of latex rubber, although they can be made of animal intestines. Only latex rubber condoms protect against disease, however. Some condoms contain a spermicide (e.g., nonoynol) that immobilizes and kills the sperm, providing additional contraception. You can get extra protection by using a foam that contains spermicide, along with the condom.

The *male condom* should be applied just before intercourse, when the man's penis is erect, before he touches the sexual partner's genitals. When the penis is being withdrawn, the condom should always be held at the base so that there is less risk of spillage, leakage, or tears (see Fig. 1.14 A and B). Effectiveness is reduced if the condom tears during intercourse. If a leak or tear occurs, use a spermicidal jelly or foam as soon as possible.

The *female condom* is made of polyurethane, a

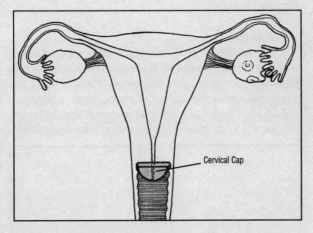

Figure 1.13 Cervical Cap
Similar to the diaphragm, the cervical cap is a small, cup-shaped, rubber device. Also used with spermicide, it is inserted into the vagina and pushed onto the cervix, where it is held in place by suction. The cap is somewhat more difficult to learn to place correctly than the diaphragm, but many women like it because it can be left in place longer and, for some, may be more comfortable.

thin but strong material that resists tearing during use. It consists of two flexible rings connected by a loose-fitting sheath. One of the rings is used to insert the condom and hold it inside the vagina. The other ring remains outside and covers the woman's labia and the base of the penis during intercourse. The female condom is prelubricated and lines the vagina after insertion (see Fig. 1.15). It is designed for one-time use only. One advantage of the female condom is that it can be inserted several hours before sex. Its fairly high failure rate is often due to incorrect use. Used properly, the female condom is nearly as effective as other techniques.

Sponge

The sponge is available without a prescription; it is made of polyurethane and contains a spermicide. Before intercourse, the sponge is inserted into the vagina to cover the cervix, forming both a physical shield and chemical barrier to sperm. It should be left in place for at least 6 hours after intercourse. The

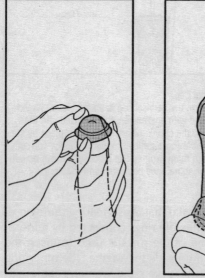
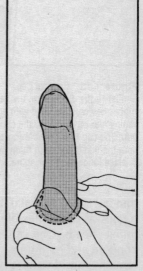

Figure 1.14 Male Condom
The male condom is one of the most widely used forms of contraception. It also offers protection against sexually transmitted diseases, including HIV, the virus that causes AIDS. The rolled-up condom is placed over the man's erect penis (A) and then unrolled downward (B). A small space is left at the tip of the condom to catch the man's semen during ejaculation.

sponge may be left in place up to 24 hours, and it is effective if intercourse is repeated during that time. As with diaphragms or condoms that contain spermicide, a small percentage of users may experience irritation or allergic reactions.

Intrauterine Devices

There are currently two types of intrauterine devices (IUD) available. One is a plastic device shaped like the letter *T* that is wound with copper, and the other

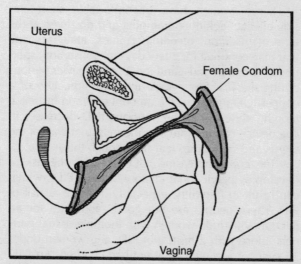

Figure 1.15 Female Condom
The newest form of barrier contraception, the female condom, also offers women protection against sexually transmitted diseases. It consists of a long rubber sheath with a closed ring at one end and a slightly larger, open ring at the other. The closed end is inserted into the vagina and fits over the cervix, like the diaphragm. The open end hangs outside the vagina, so that the interior of the vagina and the cervix are covered.

is a device that releases the hormone progesterone. When placed inside the uterus, the IUD causes an inflammatory reaction in the uterine lining that prevents pregnancy.

The IUD device must be put in place by a trained physician or nurse. It is inserted through the cervix into the uterus. Threads hang through the cervix and must be checked monthly after each period to be sure the IUD is still in place (see Fig. 1.16). The IUD containing progesterone should be replaced every year, while the copper-containing IUD can be used for 8 years.

Some women have uncomfortable short-term side effects, including cramping and dizziness at the time of insertion; bleeding, cramps, and backache that may continue for a few days after insertion; spotting between periods; and longer and heavier periods during the first few cycles after insertion. Use of a copper IUD increases the amount of blood lost each month, while use of the hormone IUD decreases it. The device can migrate into the muscular wall of the uterus and sometimes tear it, although this is rare.

The copper-releasing IUD increases the risk of developing pelvic inflammatory disease (PID), which can result in infertility, especially in those at risk of PID. These people are not good candidates for an IUD; they include women with multiple sexual partners, those with a history of PID, and women under 25 years of age who have not had children. An IUD is a good choice for women who have completed their families and are in monogamous sexual relationships.

Periodic Abstinence
Also known as natural family planning or the rhythm method, periodic abstinence relies on close observa-

tion of a woman's cycle to detect when ovulation occurs. Women using this method note the temperature increase that occurs just before ovulation and the change in cervical mucus from dry to wet and slippery that occurs around the same time. It takes into account the fact that sperm live an average of 5 days in the uterus and that the lifespan of the egg after ovulation is 1–3 days. In general, a couple should not have sexual intercourse 7 days before and 3 days after ovulation. Couples who use this method should obtain detailed instructions about it and follow the

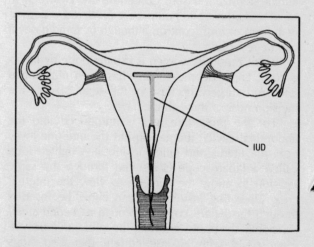

Figure 1.16   IUD
The intrauterine device (IUD) is a small, plastic device that is inserted into the uterus and left in place to prevent pregnancy. The two forms of IUD currently available are a T-shaped device wound with fine copper wire (shown here) and one containing the hormone progesterone.

plan carefully. If used perfectly, this method can be very effective. It is less effective than other forms of birth control, however, because of the difficulty in predicting exactly when ovulation will occur.

Sterilization

Men and women who no longer wish to have children may choose to undergo sterilization. The technique for women is known as tubal ligation, and the one for men is called vasectomy. The procedure for male sterilization is less risky and less expensive than female sterilization (see "Conditions and Disorders in Men"). Sterilization should be considered a permanent form of birth control, although in some cases it can be reversed.

Sterilization in women is usually done by laparoscopy. Laparoscopic surgery has been nicknamed Band-Aid surgery because of the small size of the incision near or through the navel.

For the procedure, gas is introduced into the abdominal cavity; the gas pushes the intestine away from the uterus and fallopian tubes. A lighted tube called a laparoscope is inserted through the same incision to allow the surgeon to view the internal area. Operating instruments can either be inserted through the laparoscope or through a second small incision at the pubic hair line. The fallopian tubes are then sealed with electric current that also stops bleeding. In some cases, a ring or clip can be inserted over the tubes through the laparoscope to seal them (see Fig. 1.17). Other reversible means of sealing the tubes are being explored.

The procedure is very effective in preventing pregnancy. Complications are rare but include injuries to the bowel or blood vessels and infection.

Abortion

The medical term for termination of a pregnancy by any cause is *abortion*. The term *spontaneous abortion* describes a natural end of the pregnancy, also called a miscarriage, before the fetus is able to live outside the uterus (about the first 6 months of pregnancy). If a spontaneous abortion is incomplete—if some tissue is retained in the uterus—a medical procedure may be required to be sure the uterus has been emptied and there is no risk of infection. An *elective abortion* refers to the surgical or medical termination of a pregnancy. When a woman is ill and cannot withstand the strain of the pregnancy, termination may be called therapeutic abortion.

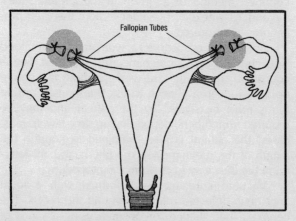

Figure 1.17 Tubal Ligation
Sterilization is a permanent form of birth control. In women, it is done by a procedure called tubal ligation, in which both fallopian tubes are cut and sealed by tying, banding, or clipping the cut ends. The egg released each month by one of the ovaries thus cannot be reached by the man's sperm.

With any form of abortion, the initial step is confirming the pregnancy. Most commercially available pregnancy tests inform you of your pregnancy status at the time of the first missed menstrual period. Although this usually occurs about 2 weeks after conception, some women have a lighter period and are unaware they are pregnant until they miss the next period, approximately 6 weeks after the date of conception.

Elective abortions can be performed in a physician's office as early as 1–2 weeks after a missed menstrual period. Using the menstrual extraction technique, the contents of the uterus are removed with a syringe. After 7 weeks of pregnancy, doctors use a procedure called vacuum curettage, the most common method of abortion in the United States. Beyond 13 weeks of pregnancy, more involved procedures are required.

Before the procedure, a woman has her blood type checked and a pregnancy test repeated. She is counseled by health care workers about the procedure and given a chance to ask questions. Consent forms must be signed by the patient and may be required from others, depending on state law. In most cases, the patient is also examined to confirm the length of the pregnancy so the physician can determine the best way to perform the procedure.

Vacuum curettage is performed with a local anesthetic, injected into and around the cervix. The cervix is then dilated, or opened, using a series of gradually larger metal rods or a synthetic material that swells. The contents of the uterus are then removed with a suction device. As the uterus contracts to its previous size, some cramping may result. The amount of blood lost is usually small. In most clinics, only about 1 percent of women have complications, such as infection, perforation of the uterus, or bleeding.

Abortions in later stages have a higher risk of complications and should be performed in a hospital or a specialized clinic. They can be done with suction or by administering agents that bring on labor. In some extreme cases, surgery may be required.

A drug called mifepristone can induce abortion; it is also known as the French pill, or RU–486 and is not currently available in this country. Efforts are ongoing to have this drug available so it can be offered as a safer, nonsurgical approach to abortion.

In the days when abortions were outlawed, women sought abortions from unlicensed providers who frequently did not use sterile techniques and who did not monitor women for complications. As a result, women developed advanced infections that spread from the uterus to the bloodstream and the abdominal cavity. Such infections could result in permanent sterility or death. Today, abortions are extremely safe when performed in a proper medical setting by a licensed practitioner. An abortion has no effect on a woman's ability to have children in the future.

Cancer Detection

When cancer develops in a woman's reproductive organs, it is rarely accompanied by symptoms. (See Fig. 1.18). In some cases, cancer can be prevented by detecting precancerous changes in the cells. In others, noncancerous conditions can cause symptoms that must be explored to rule out cancer.

Although the initial evaluation can be done by a gynecologist, a gynecologic oncologist, who specializes in cancer of the reproductive organs, should provide care once cancer is diagnosed. The earlier cancer is detected and treated, the better the chance for cure.

Cervix

The Pap test can detect changes in the cells of the cervix that are not cancer but may warn that cancer could develop (see Fig. 1.10). Some of these changes return to normal on their own, whereas for others, treatment can keep cancer from developing. The Pap test can allow almost all cases of cervical cancer to be prevented, which is why it is so important that you have one regularly.

There are virtually no symptoms during the earliest stage of cervical cancer. The most common early warning signs of cervical cancer are spotting or irregular bleeding or bleeding after intercourse. These signs should prompt an immediate visit to a gynecologist.

Risk factors for cervical cancer include early age at first intercourse, having multiple sexual partners, smoking, and infection with human papillomavirus (HPV). Because HPV is spread through sexual contact, the risk factors for contacting this virus include having multiple male sexual partners, who themselves have had multiple sexual partners. Women are most at risk during the teenage years when cervical cells are maturing.

In the Pap test, cells of the cervix are examined under a microscope to detect abnormalities (see Fig. 1.19). The results are reported in categories developed by the National Cancer Institute, called the Bethesda System, and treated accordingly:

- Normal: No abnormal cells are present.

- Atypical Squamous Cells of Undetermined Significance (ASCUS): These cells appear abnormal, but it is not clear exactly what that may mean. Although some doctors may believe that further testing is needed, in most cases these changes can be assessed by repeat Pap tests at 3–6 month intervals, preferably not during menstruation. If results are normal in two consecu-

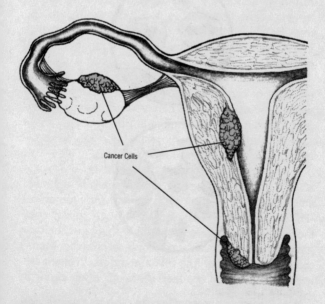

Cancer Cells

Figure 1.18 Cancer
Possible sites of cancer in women include the ovary, uterus, and cervix.

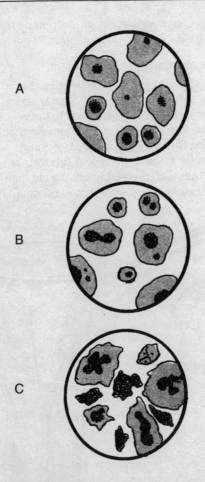

Figure 1.19 Pap Test
In the Pap test, cells collected from the cervix are examined under a microscope to detect abnormalities. Shown here are normal cervical cells (A), cells showing cervical dysplasia (B), and typical cancer cells (C).

tive tests, annual Pap tests can be resumed and no further treatment is needed. About 70 percent of patients with results in this category need no further treatment.

- Low-Grade Squamous Intraepithelial Lesions: Includes changes seen with HPV infection as well as early precancerous changes, also called mild dysplasia or cervical intraepithelial neoplasia grade 1 (CIN 1). About 60 percent of these changes go away on their own, and about 15 percent go on to a more advanced stage. Follow-up may involve monitoring the condition with Pap tests at 3–6-month intervals and performing a procedure called colposcopy (see "Procedures") if the condition persists.

- High-Grade Squamous Intraepithelial Lesions: Includes moderate and severe dysplasia (CIN 2 and 3) as well as carcinoma in situ, which is a severe form of precancer. A sample of the tissue is obtained by biopsying the most severe area to confirm the types of abnormalities seen through the colposcope. The affected areas are then removed with local surgery using various techniques: loop electrosurgical excision procedure (LEEP), laser, freezing techniques, or electrosurgery (see "Procedures"). A procedure called cervical conization may be performed to remove a cone-shaped wedge from the cervix.

- Invasive Cancer: Early stage invasive cancer can be treated with either radical hysterectomy (removal of the uterus) or radiation therapy. In later stages, especially when the lymph nodes are involved, a combination of surgery, radiation, and possibly chemotherapy may be used.

There is a 90 percent likelihood that the treatment for early precancerous changes will completely remove any abnormal tissue. About 10 percent of women have an abnormal Pap smear during that first year after treatment. Treatment of this persistent area has a cure rate of about 90 percent. Thus, there is about a 99 percent cure rate with two treatments. Women who have been treated should continue to have yearly Pap tests, however, even after menopause or hysterectomy.

Uterus

Cancer of the lining of the uterus, the endometrium, is the most common gynecologic cancer. About 31,000 cases occur annually. The survival rate for this cancer is high if the cancer is diagnosed in a very early stage.

The most frequent symptom of endometrial cancer is spotting or irregular bleeding, which should alert a woman to seek treatment. Women in the menopausal years should consult their physicians immediately if they develop spotting after their regular periods have stopped for 1 year or more.

The greatest risk factor for endometrial cancer appears to be excess amounts of the hormone estrogen. Estrogen stimulates the uterine lining to grow, causing a condition called endometrial hyperplasia, a form of precancer. The excess estrogen can come from a variety of sources:

■ Hormone replacement therapy taken during and after menopause includes estrogen and progesterone. If estrogen is taken alone, a woman's risk of developing endometrial cancer is increased. By taking both estrogen and progesterone pills, however, a woman's risk of cancer is even lower than those who take no therapy.

■ Fat cells are the most abundant source of excess estrogen production. Some fat cells normally convert inactive adrenal hormones into very active estrogenlike hormones. These hormones overstimulate the uterine lining to grow, possibly out of control, into cancer. Women who are slightly overweight have a 3-fold risk of developing endometrial cancer and those who are nearly twice their recommended weight have a 10-fold risk of developing endometrial cancer.

The diagnosis is confirmed by performing a uterine biopsy to obtain a sample of the lining to study. This procedure can be performed in a physician's office, without any anesthesia. The "D&C," or dilation and curettage, is rarely needed now that suction biopsies can be done in the office.

Treatment usually consists of a hysterectomy. The ovaries are usually removed (oophorectomy), along with the lymph nodes. A careful search is made for any sign of further spread (see "Staging of Endometrial Cancer"). A general gynecologist can perform the surgery in early stage cancer but a gynecologic oncologist should always be available if advanced disease is found during the surgery. If advanced disease is diagnosed preoperatively, the gynecologic oncologist should perform the surgery. After surgery and complete pathological evaluation of the uterus, the ovaries, and the lymph nodes, further treatment may be recommended in the form of either radiation or chemotherapy.

STAGING OF ENDOMETRIAL CANCER

Stage I   Cancer confined to the body of the uterus.

Stage II   Cancer extended from the body of the uterus to the cervix.

Stage III Cancer spread out to lymph nodes or onto the ovaries.

Stage IV   Distant spread to the lung or into the bladder or rectum.

Ovarian Cancer

Ovarian cancer is the most malignant of all of the gynecologic cancers. Approximately 24,000 women develop ovarian cancer each year, and unfortunately many are not diagnosed until the cancer is in advanced stages. The risk factors for ovarian cancer include advanced age, not having children or having them late in life, and a family history of ovarian cancer or other cancers such as breast or colon cancers.

Ovarian cancer gives only vague early warning signs, such as a change in bowel pattern, a feeling of bloating, or simply pelvic discomfort. These symptoms may be due to pressure from a pelvic mass or tumor implants on the bowel wall.

When ovarian cancer grows, some women think they are only getting fat and don't investigate the cause of the swelling. The cancer can cause fluid to accumulate within the abdominal cavity, causing the abdomen to swell. This fluid contains cancer cells and can spread even into the lung cavity, where more fluid can accumulate.

Since there are so few warning signs in the early stages, this cancer is usually diagnosed later, when tumor nodules from the ovaries extend to the surface of the liver, the bowel, the stomach, or inside the abdominal wall. Cancer is often suspected by pelvic exam and confirmed by ultrasound. A blood test also can be performed to measure a substance called CA–125 that circulates in the blood. CA–125 is used as a tumor marker because levels are increased when tumors are present. Because levels are increased by the presence of many other benign disorders, this test is not used to screen healthy women.

Therapy usually begins with surgery to remove all the tumor, followed by chemotherapy. The chemotherapy is fairly effective at removing any tumor cells left after surgery. While a complete cure of this cancer occurs in only about 20–30 percent of women, chemotherapy usually prolongs life very significantly.

Ovarian Cysts

Often a cyst may develop on an ovary. This fluid-filled growth is not cancerous in most cases. Some may be the earliest sign that a cancer has formed, however, so all ovarian cysts should be taken seriously and evaluated. Ovarian cysts may have no symptoms; large cysts can cause a feeling of pelvic pressure or fullness. Diagnosis is usually by vaginal ultrasound: A small probe is passed into the vagina that reveals details of the ovaries and uterus. The CA–125 blood test can also be performed to assess the likelihood of ovarian cancer. Treatment of ovarian cysts ranges from careful monitoring of simple small cysts to surgical removal of any ovarian cysts that may suggest a malignancy. Oral contraceptives do not make an ovarian cyst disappear any faster. If you have an ovarian cyst that is under observation, your doctor should check it again within three months to make sure it has not changed or grown larger. Always get a second opinion before having surgery for an ovarian cyst.

Vagina

Cancer of the vagina that does not involve the vulva or the cervix is rare. One form is caused by exposure to a drug called diethylstilbestrol, or DES, in women whose mothers took the drug while they were pregnant. In the early 1950s DES was prescribed to women who were at risk of losing their pregnancies. Now, their daughters are at risk for some cancers of the vagina. A registry has been created to keep track of these women so they can receive careful monitoring. The cancer usually develops around age 19; treatment is by hysterectomy, and it has a 90 percent cure rate if identified in the earliest stage of growth.

Vulva

Vulvar cancer is a rare gynecologic malignancy. It almost always strikes women who are in the menopausal years and appears to be linked to infection with HPV. The cancer appears as a small sore or small lump on one of the outer lips of the vulva. Sometimes it can itch, but it usually does not cause any pain. Many women delay seeing their gynecologists, hoping the sore will disappear; however, this delay allows for continued tumor growth. If you have a small sore, lump, or ulcer on any area of the vulva that is new and does not go away within a week, see your physician.

The diagnosis is based on the results of a biopsy, in which the area is numbed and a small amount of tissue is removed to be studied. If the cancer is found in early stages, surgery is performed. Usually, the area of cancer must be removed with a rim of normal tissue of approximately 1 inch in diameter all the way around the cancer. This is called a radical partial vulvectomy. In most stages of disease, lymph nodes in the groin should also be removed. If cancer has spread to the lymph nodes, radiation therapy is usually required.

Ectopic Pregnancy

Normally, once the egg is fertilized in the fallopian tubes, it travels to the uterus and becomes implanted there. When, for any reason, the fertilized egg implants anywhere else along the route, the pregnancy is said to be ectopic, or in the wrong place (see Fig. 1.20).

Ectopic pregnancy occurs when the opening of the fallopian tube is twisted or narrowed, due to scar tissue formed by infection or surgery. The passage of the fertilized egg to the uterus is blocked, and the egg begins to develop within the fallopian tube lining, on the surface of the ovary, or within the abdominal or pelvic cavity. The egg can only develop for a few weeks before its growth is hindered by the size of the fallopian tube.

In an ectopic pregnancy, symptoms of early pregnancy, an abnormally light period, and pelvic pain can occur. Many women have no symptoms until the pregnancy causes a rupture of the fallopian tube or there is bleeding from a nearby blood vessel. This causes severe abdominal pain, shock, and collapse—a medical emergency of the first order.

If you have a history of tubal infections or previous ectopic pregnancy and suspect you are pregnant, you should be carefully monitored by your physician to be sure that the pregnancy is within the uterus. Ectopic pregnancy is diagnosed by doing tests to measure hormone levels that indicate pregnancy. Once pregnancy has been confirmed, ultrasound can determine its location and size.

If the fallopian tube has ruptured, ectopic pregnancy is an emergency that requires surgery to remove the pregnancy and control bleeding. In some cases, the tube can then be rejoined. Many surgeons are now performing this procedure through the laparoscope. Conservative surgery in which the fallopian tube is simply opened and the pregnancy lifted out is frequently possible and conserves the tube, and thus your ability to have children. Another procedure for small, early ectopic pregnancies involves the intramuscular injection of chemotherapy; the usual result is loss of the pregnancy in about 7 days.

Endometriosis

The tissue that lines the inside of the uterus responds to hormones that cause it to thicken and bleed each month. This tissue can also grow outside the uterus, on the pelvic organs. When this occurs, these areas

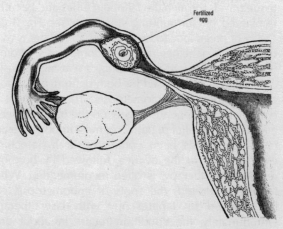

Figure 1.20   Ectopic Pregnancy
In an ectopic pregnancy, the fertilized ovum becomes attached in a
place other than inside the uterus. Most ectopic pregnancies occur
in a fallopian tube.

can become inflamed and sometimes painful, and
scar tissue develops.

Some women with endometriosis, even severe
endometriosis, have no symptoms. Others can have
intense pain, especially when the endometrial tissue
is shed into the pelvic area during the menstrual period. The pain can be felt throughout the entire area or
may be confined to the uterus. Pain usually appears
only during the menstrual period, but can start just
before and gradually increase until bleeding starts,
usually easing after up to 72 hours. In addition to
pelvic pain, endometriosis is a common cause of
infertility because it causes the fallopian tubes to mal-
function.

Researchers have not been able to pinpoint causes of endometriosis. One theory is that endometrial

tissue travels through the fallopian tubes and becomes implanted on surrounding structures (see Fig. 1.21). Delay of pregnancy to beyond age 30 or later is associated with a higher risk of endometriosis. Women who have never had a pregnancy are at highest risk.

Laparoscopy is used for both definitive diagnosis and treatment of endometriosis. The treatment of endometriosis depends largely on the patient's needs and desires. If relief of pain is of most importance and childbearing has been completed, a hysterectomy with removal of the ovaries, followed by hormone replacement therapy, is often recommended. When fertility is desired, the spots of endometriosis can be removed by laparoscopy with laser therapy. Unfortunately, the condition recurs in about one-third of women treated.

Synthetic hormones can be used to shrink the endometriosis implants, but the effect is temporary. The implants usually return to their premedication level within a few months after treatment ends. Treatment can be given for only 6 months because it decreases the estrogen level. This brief remission of the disease can be time enough to allow conception soon after, if that is desired. Because prevention of ovulation can reduce the discomfort, many women take oral contraceptives. However, some still have pain and require surgery for relief.

Fibroids

Benign fibrous growths of the uterine wall are called fibroids. Some fibroids bulge outward from the wall; others extend from the uterine surface on a stalk. A fibroid can also extend into the uterine lining, com-

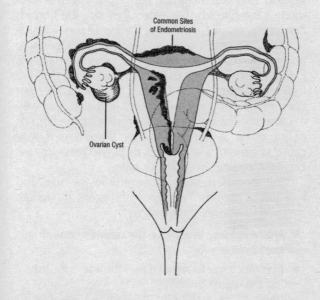

Figure 1.21 Endometriosis
Endometriosis is a condition in which tissue similar to that lining the uterus is present outside the uterus. It may be attached to the outside of the uterus, ovaries, or tubes, or it may be present in other areas of the abdomen.

pressing the endometrium or forming a growth on a stem within the endometrial cavity. About 20 percent of women of reproductive age have fibroids, and for most of them the fibroids pose no problem.

Fibroids enlarge the uterus and can cause pressure and discomfort in the pelvis, however. Internal uterine fibroids can also compress the endometrial lining and cause excessive bleeding during and occasionally between menstrual periods. Younger women rarely have fibroids, but when they do, the fibroids can press against the lining of the uterus causing infertility. The most serious complication is pressure and blockage of the ureters, the tubes draining the kidneys. On rare occasions, a fibroid can develop into a malignant tumor. Fibroids have been the most common reason for hysterectomy in the past, as well as currently. The only reason for removing the fibroids or for doing a hysterectomy for fibroids is if they cause symptoms like bladder or pelvic pressure, excessive bleeding, infertility, or pain.

Ultrasound is used to determine the size and location of fibroids. Two types of surgery, if needed, are used to remove the growths:

- Hysterectomy to remove the uterus and with it, the fibroids
- Myomectomy to remove the fibroids only, leaving the uterus intact

The selection of the type of surgery used rests with the woman and her surgeon. For a woman who wants to maintain her fertility, a myomectomy is the treatment of choice. It might also be preferred by the woman who wishes to have her uterus and ovaries left intact.

Myomectomy usually involves more blood loss than a hysterectomy, because the fibroid can have a rich blood supply. During a hysterectomy, the location of each blood vessel that feeds the uterus is well known and can be clamped off so that little bleeding occurs. During myomectomy, the blood supply to the fibroid is less clearly defined and blood loss can be heavy. Many gynecologists recommend that women who do not want to retain fertility simply have the top half or the entire uterus removed in what is called a partial hysterectomy.

Sometimes this procedure can be made easier by shrinking the fibroid prior to surgery. This is done by prescribing hormones that mimic menopause and decrease the amount of estrogens, resulting in shrinkage of the fibroid by as much as 50 percent.

Women can usually become pregnant after removal of a fibroid and carry the pregnancy to full term, although they may occasionally require a caesarean delivery.

Menopause

At menopause, a woman stops menstruating and her ovaries no longer produce estrogen. The average age at the last menstrual period is 51. This natural process begins several years before, as a woman's ovaries produce less and less estrogen. The lack of estrogen can produce a number of effects:

- Hot flashes or flushes can occur. These are sudden feelings of heat that spread over the body, often accompanied by a flushed face and sweating. They appear at any time without warning and are most troublesome at night when they can interfere with sleep.

- Vaginal tissues may become dryer, thinner, and less flexible. This can result in painful intercourse, urinary tract problems, or sagging of pelvic organs because the tissues that support them lose their elasticity.

- Osteoporosis, or bone loss can cause bones to become thin and brittle. Supplemental estrogen can help guard against it, as can a diet high in calcium, regular exercise, and stopping smoking.

- Cardiovascular disease becomes more of a risk for women after menopause because estrogen no longer gives them natural protection from heart attack and stroke.

- Emotional changes, such as mood swings, irritability, and depression can accompany menopause, but these symptoms are more likely related to insomnia caused by hot flashes at night than to the lack of estrogen.

Not all women have all of these symptoms and they are not always long lasting. You can continue to have a full and healthy life for many years beyond menopause. Some of the symptoms of menopause can be eased through diet and exercise. Others can be relieved by replacing the estrogen no longer produced by the ovaries. Hormone replacement therapy can relieve the symptoms of menopause, in addition to lowering the risk of heart disease and osteoporosis.

Estrogen is given along with the hormone progestin (a synthetic version of the natural hormone progesterone) to protect against endometrial cancer, a risk when estrogen is taken alone. Estrogen by itself causes the lining of the uterus to overgrow and increases the risk of cancer of the endometrium. Progestin is taken with estrogen to oppose it and keep the lining of the endometrium in check. In fact, taking progestin with estrogen actually lowers the risk of cancer to less than that of a woman not taking hormone therapy.

Estrogen is processed through the liver and

affects the levels of cholesterol. Estrogen increases high-density cholesterol (the good cholesterol) and lowers low-density cholesterol (the bad cholesterol), thus reducing the risk of heart disease. Without estrogen, a woman's risk of heart disease approaches that of a man by age 65.

Women are at higher risk of osteoporosis because they have less bone mass than men to begin with and because they tend to have less calcium stored in their bones. Thus, when they lose the protective effect of estrogen, the natural process of bone loss speeds up so they are losing bone faster than it is being replaced.

Osteoporosis and cardiovascular disease do not have symptoms in their early stages as they are conditions that develop over time. Hormone replacement therapy to prevent symptoms of menopause also helps prevent these conditions. To provide long-term protection, the therapy must be taken long term.

Hormone replacement therapy is not for everyone. It is not recommended for women who have had breast cancer, endometrial cancer, or liver cancer. The link between breast cancer and hormone replacement therapy is still not clear. There may be a slight increase in a woman's chance of developing breast cancer if she has been taking hormones for more than 15 years.

Hormone replacement therapy can have other side effects. The progestin causes monthly bleeding or spotting, which can be unexpected and bothersome. Other side effects include breast tenderness, fluid retention, swelling, mood changes, and pelvic cramping. Because of the side effects, some women choose to take estrogen alone. These women should be monitored carefully for abnormal bleeding. Their doctors may suggest that an endometrial biopsy be performed so a small amount of tissue can be examined.

Women who prefer not to take hormone replacement therapy can obtain relief of symptoms and help prevent bone loss and heart disease in other ways. To facilitate decisions about hormones, women should have a fasting cholesterol and a bone density test. Estrogen cream, used in the vagina, can treat vaginal dryness. A balanced diet rich in calcium and low in fat, regular exercise, and avoiding alcohol and tobacco can help reduce the rate of bone loss and protect against heart disease. Regardless of age or whether they are taking hormone replacement therapy, women should continue to have regular pelvic exams, mammograms, and Pap tests after they reach menopause.

Menstrual Problems

Most women experience some discomfort with their menstrual periods. Certain conditions, such as endometriosis or fibroids, can increase pain during menstrual periods. Any severe pain, unusual spotting or bleeding, or missed menstrual periods could be a sign of a problem that requires medical attention.

Amenorrhea

Amenorrhea is the absence of menstruation. This absence is normal before puberty, after menopause, and during pregnancy. Primary amenorrhea occurs when a woman reaches the age of 18 and has never had a period. It is usually caused by a problem in the endocrine system that regulates hormones. Secondary amenorrhea is present when a woman has had regular periods that stop for longer than 12 months. Amenorrhea may be triggered by a wide range of events:

Primary amenorrhea

- Ovarian failure
- Problems in the nervous system or the pituitary gland in the endocrine system that affect maturation at puberty
- Birth defects in which the reproductive structures do not develop properly

Secondary amenorrhea

- Problems that affect estrogen levels, such as stress, weight loss, exercise, or illness
- Problems affecting the pituitary, thyroid, or adrenal gland
- Ovarian tumors or surgical removal of the ovaries

To diagnose and treat amenorrhea it may be necessary to consult a reproductive endocrinologist. Treatment is based on the problem diagnosed. Blood tests are usually performed and many patients are asked to keep a record of their early morning temperatures to detect the rise in temperature that occurs with ovulation.

Cramps

The sensation of spasmodic cramping or a feeling of chronic achy fullness can occur with a normal menstrual cycle and a normal anatomy. The pain is due to uterine contractions, caused by substances called prostaglandins.

Prostaglandins circulate within the blood. They can cause diarrhea by speeding up the contractions of the intestinal tract and lower blood pressure by relaxing the muscles of blood vessels. Thus many women frequently notice that severe menstrual pain is associated with mild diarrhea and occasionally an overall sensation of faintness in which they become pale, sweaty, and sometimes nauseated. Some women actually have fainting spells because of the low blood pressure resulting from the action of prostaglandins.

To relieve cramps, your doctor may recommend drugs called prostaglandin inhibitors or nonsteroidal anti-inflammatory drugs (NSAIDs), which are available without a prescription. Taking medication immediately at the onset of any symptoms usually results in dramatic improvement or complete relief. Taking these drugs even before symptoms begin may help, too. Relief also may be obtained by applications of heat and mild exercise.

Excessive Bleeding

Some women experience a menopause characterized by irregular, unpredictable, often heavy bleeding. If you develop severe irregular bleeding as you approach menopause, or experience new bleeding a year after your final period, your doctor should do a biopsy to confirm that no precancerous changes have taken place. This biopsy does not need to be the traditional dilation and curettage (D&C) that is performed in a hospital under general anesthesia. Rather, the biopsy is a simple procedure that takes place in the doctor's office. A slender, soft, plastic canula is inserted through the cervix and a small sample of uterine tissue is obtained. The cost of this biopsy is about 10 percent of the cost of a regular D&C and provides the same information. These tests are 99.5 percent reliable in diagnosing a precancerous condition or cancer, if present. If there is no sign of cancer, excessive bleeding can be treated with hormone therapy or surgery on the lining of the uterus.

Pelvic Inflammatory Disease

Infection with the STDs chlamydia and gonorrhea can lead to pelvic inflammatory disease (PID). In PID, infection spreads upward through the cervix, the uterus, and the fallopian tubes into the pelvic cavity. White blood cells battling the infection cause a pus-like discharge to surround the ovaries. The body tries to wall off this infection by creating filmy adhesions (a fibrous wall) from organ to organ to limit the spread of the infection. The adhesions can distort the fallopian tubes and result in infertility.

Early symptoms of PID include pelvic pain associated with fever and weakness; there also may be a vaginal discharge. If the infection continues, an abscess can form within the pelvis. The typical PID attack strikes after a menstrual period and begins with pelvic pain. Motion, even walking, can be painful. If the abscess develops, it can send bacteria into the blood stream, causing high fever, chills, joint infections, and even death.

Diagnosis usually is based on the symptoms and presence of the abscess. In some cases, a sample of the discharge from the abscess can be used to identify the organism causing the infection. Antibiotics can stop the infection before an abscess has formed, if treatment is started early. If the infection is severe, some patients may require intravenous antibiotics in a hospital setting. Surgery may be necessary to drain an abscess, but it is usually not necessary to remove the uterus, tubes, and ovaries.

Premenstrual Syndrome

The regular, recurring symptoms that occur just prior to menstruation are called premenstrual syndrome (PMS). PMS is not a disease but rather a collection of symptoms that disappear once the menstrual period has begun.

Nearly all menstruating women experience a set of symptoms that tell them their periods are coming. For some women, these symptoms can be quite severe, involving a combination of emotional and physical changes. Emotional changes may include anger, anxiety, confusion, mood swings, tension, crying, depression, and an inability to concentrate. Physical symptoms include bloating, swollen breasts, fatigue, constipation, headache, and clumsiness.

The diagnosis rests on confirming the cyclic nature of these symptoms and ruling out any underlying psychological or physical dysfunction. Many women are asked to chart their symptoms so they can be related to the menstrual cycle to detect a pattern. The symptoms usually occur about 7 days before a menstrual period and go away once it begins.

The cause of PMS is unknown, despite extensive research into abnormal types of hormones that are secreted at this time, unusual ratios of one hormone to another, and imbalance between sodium and body water retention. Many theories have been studied, but none has been shown to be the primary cause. As a result, the condition is difficult to treat.

Treatment is generally aimed at relieving symptoms. Keeping a calendar and being aware of when symptoms occur helps most women; simply knowing their distressing symptoms are related to the onset of their periods can have a calming effect. There are other things you can try to ease symptoms of PMS:

- Dietary changes provide relief for some women: Decreasing sodium, sugar, caffeine, and alcohol; increasing complex carbohydrates; and eating smaller, more frequent meals.

- Dietary supplementation of calcium, magnesium, and vitamins B_6 and E may reduce symptions.

- Exercise has been shown to help in depression and, theoretically, may be of some benefit for PMS.

- Diuretics can relieve the feeling of bloating and swelling caused by fluid retention.

- Pain can be relieved with nonsteroidal anti-inflammatory drugs (NSAIDs).

- Oral contraceptives are helpful in relieving symptoms in some women.

■ Severe breast tenderness can be relieved by taking bromocriptine, a drug that stops the production of certain hormones, but this drug does not help other PMS symptoms.

Many medications have been tried with limited success. Some of them are expensive and most have side effects. It may be necessary to combine some remedies on a trial and error basis, along with modifications in diet and exercise.

Rape

Rape is sexual intercourse by force; it is epidemic in our country. This violent crime has both psychological as well as medical aspects that affect women's health.

A rape should be reported within 48 hours of its occurrence, as crucial evidence of it is more difficult to obtain after that time. Women should not wash, bathe, urinate, defecate, drink, or take any medication prior to reporting a rape. A practitioner experienced in this area should perform a thorough exam so there is evidence available if charges are brought against the accused rapist.

A physician first asks the woman to describe what happened, and then examines her clothing for damage, taking particular note if there are any materials such as soil or stains such as body fluids sticking to the clothing. The physician next asks if any drugs or alcohol were taken by the woman or the rapist, because this may become an important issue during court procedures.

The physical exam consists of looking for evidence on the whole body, even though not every woman who has been raped has been physically injured. The physician measures and charts all injuries and may photograph them, looking carefully for bite marks, bruises, grip marks, and scratches. Samples are taken of the vaginal fluid to check for infection or sperm. Mouth swabs and saliva samples are obtained to look for bacteria and semen and possibly to perform DNA studies of the sample. Urine samples may be obtained to determine whether drugs were involved. Blood samples are obtained to test for HIV as well as hepatitis. If the HIV test is negative, another HIV test should be done in 6 months to determine whether the virus was contracted during the rape. A woman may be given treatment against possible STDs, and she should be offered emergency contraception if there is a chance pregnancy could result from the assault.

After the exam, comfort, support, and counseling are key to complete recovery. There are many groups available to counsel women who are recovering from previous molestation or rape.

Vaginitis

The internal environment of the vagina consists of a delicate balance of organisms that, along with normal vaginal secretions, keep it healthy and clean. When that balance is disrupted by either an infection, a health problem, or some type of irritation, vaginitis can occur. Bacteria or yeast that grows normally in the vagina can overgrow and cause itching, redness, and pain in the vaginal area. Infections from other organisms, as well as allergic reactions, can also cause vaginitis.

Any new discharge accompanied by an odor, or abnormal itching, could be a sign of a vaginal infection. The characteristics of the discharge—its color, odor, and amount—can be a clue to the cause. Yeast is the most common cause of vaginitis, but bacteria and parasites can also cause it. The cause of vaginitis must be identified for treatment to be effective.

Bacterial Vaginosis

Among the more common vaginal infections, bacterial vaginosis is caused by the *Gardnerella, Bacteriodes,* and *Peptostreptococcus* bacteria. The primary symptom is a foul-smelling, profuse, watery vaginal discharge.

The diagnosis is confirmed by microscopic examination of the discharge. Treatment for this infection is the antibiotic metronidazole. Often, the infection recurs; longer treatment may be needed to prevent recurrences.

Yeast Infection

Some women are unusually susceptible to this most common of all vaginal infections. The cause may be a recent course of antibiotics that can decrease the normal vaginal bacteria and allow for an overgrowth of yeast. Other conditions, like diabetes and HIV infection, are also associated with recurrent yeast infections.

Your doctor will want to confirm that yeast is the cause by examining the vaginal discharge under a microscope. Discuss multiple recurrent yeast infections with your physician, because other problems such as diabetes should be ruled out.

Once you can recognize the symptoms of yeast

vaginitis, you can treat yourself by purchasing any one of the over-the-counter antifungal creams or suppository preparations. Treatment is also available in pill form by prescription.

PROCEDURES FOR WOMEN

Cryotherapy

Cryotherapy involves freezing cells on the cervix to remove abnormal cells. Freezing kills cells but does not remove them from the vagina. The dead cells dissolve into the vaginal fluid and are washed away in the normal secretions. This can cause an increased vaginal discharge for about 2 weeks after the procedure.

Colposcopy

In colposcopy, the cervix, vagina, and vulva skin are examined systematically under microscopic magnification. When abnormal areas are detected, a sample is taken for further examination (a biopsy).

During the procedure, a speculum is inserted in the vagina to spread the vaginal walls, and a vinegar solution is sprayed into the cervix. The abnormal surface cells appear white, and normal cells remain pink. The entire area is examined, and a biopsy of any white area is performed.

Most women have a slight cramp for a minute or so during the biopsy. Otherwise, this procedure requires no anesthesia and is well tolerated. If a woman has severe cramps with her menstrual cycle, medication can be given before the exam to reduce discomfort.

Occasionally a scraping of tissue is obtained from the inner lining of the cervix beyond the limits of the area that can be seen. This scraping provides extra assurance that the entire abnormality has been identified. Once the biopsy results are available, therapy can be started.

Dilation and Curettage

Often referred to as a D&C, dilation and curettage removes the lining and contents of the uterus. Once the cervix is widened by dilators, the uterine lining is scraped out with a curette, a spoonlike instrument. A D&C is used to perform abortions, remove the lining of the uterus in cases of severe bleeding, or test for uterine cancer (see Fig. 1.22). A D&C is performed in a hospital or an ambulatory surgery center using general anesthetic. Rapid recovery with minimal spotting for 1 to 2 days can be expected. It has largely been replaced by the office biopsy.

Hysterectomy

A complete or total hysterectomy is removal of the entire uterus with the cervix (see Fig. 1.23A). A partial hysterectomy involves removing only a portion of the uterus (see Fig. 1.23B). A radical hysterectomy involves the removal of the uterus, cervix, lymph nodes, and other support structures around the

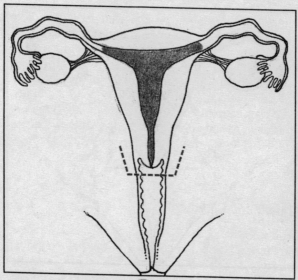

Figure 1.22.   Dilation And Curettage

Dilation and curettage (D&C) is a procedure used to remove the endometrium (the lining of the uterus) and the contents of the uterus. A speculum is inserted into the vagina, the cervix is grasped with a small tonguelike instrument, and the inside of the uterus is gently scraped out with another instrument.

cervix and uterus. (see Fig. 1.23C) A hysterectomy can be performed through the vagina or through a cut in the abdomen, depending on the reasons for the surgery.

Reasons for performing a hysterectomy should be clearly understood prior to the procedure. Following are the most common reasons for a hysterectomy:

- ■ Fibroids
- ■ Endometriosis

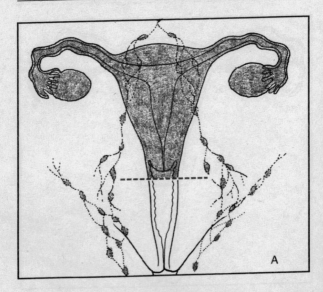

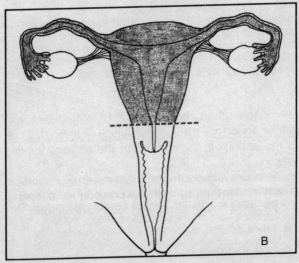

- Cancer
- Endometrial hyperplasia
- Menstrual/menopausal symptoms
- Cervical dysplasia
- Pain

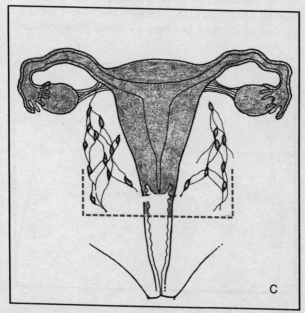

Figure 1.23 Hysterectomy

Hysterectomy, the surgical removal of the uterus, may be done in a number of ways, depending on the problem being treated. A total hysterectomy (A) involves the removal of the entire uterus, along with the ovaries and fallopian tubes. In a partial hysterectomy (B), the uterus and tubes are removed, but the ovaries and cervix are left in place. A radical hysterectomy (C) entails removal of the entire uterus, the tubes, and the ovaries, along with the lymph nodes and the support structures surrounding these organs.

A vertical incision in the lower abdomen is used for abdominal hysterectomy or for cancer or a very large fibroid. For other conditions, a horizontal incision is placed just above the pubic bone, which can be hidden in the pubic hair (see Fig. 1.24). This location results in less postoperative pain.

A vaginal hysterectomy involves less discomfort than an abdominal hysterectomy because no abdominal incision must be made. Vaginal hysterectomies

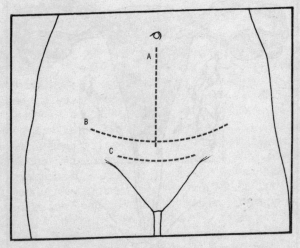

Figure 1.24 Hysterectomy Incisions
The type of incision used for a hysterectomy depends on the reason for and nature of the problem for which it is being performed. A vertical incision (A) may be used for uterine cancer or a very large fibroid. Other conditions may necessitate the use of a transverse, or horizontal, incision (B). The location and size of a transverse incision also depends on the problem being treated; a low transverse incision (C) often can be hidden in the pubic hair.

are seldom performed on women who have had no children because the ligaments are tighter and the vaginal passage is small. It is indicated when there is a small uterus, and the patient has had children, because the vagina and the connecting structures of the uterus are more pliable.

Vaginal hysterectomy is now available to more women because it can be done with a laparoscope. When the laparoscope is used, it is placed into the abdomen through a small incision in the abdominal wall. The laparoscope is a telescopelike probe that can identify the structures and cut away problems outside the uterus, such as adhesions. The uterus can then be removed through the vagina with less post-operative pain and scarring.

Recovery time varies depending on the procedure. Usually, normal activities, including sex, can be resumed in about 4–6 weeks. Until then, activities such as driving, sports, and light physical work may be increased gradually. Adhesions, or scar tissue, can develop after any surgery. They can cause pain during bowel function, intercourse, or exercise. If adhesions are particularly troublesome, laparoscopic surgery can be used to relieve them, although they may return in the future.

Very few women notice a change in their sexual sensations after hysterectomy that could be related to the functions of the uterus during sexual activity or to their own sense of loss of their uterus. For most women, however, hysterectomy has no effect on sexual satisfaction. Many women have a sense of freedom from symptoms of the condition corrected, as well as from the concern of monthly periods and potential pregnancy. If you have any doubts about having a hysterectomy, always get a second opinion.

Hysteroscopy

Hysteroscopy allows the inside of the uterus and the openings of the fallopian tubes to be viewed on a video camera or a monitor. The hysteroscope is a telescope that is inserted to look at the walls of the uterus for signs of disease or other problems (such as an IUD that has slipped out of place). It can be guided to the fallopian tubes to find any obstruction and, in some cases, remove it. Some surgical procedures can also be performed with hysteroscopy. The procedure may be performed in a doctor's office using local anesthetic.

Laparoscopy

In laparoscopy, a lighted tube with a magnifying lens on the end allows the operator to see inside the body. Laparoscopy can be used to diagnose a condition, such as endometriosis; it also can be used to perform surgery.

Laparoscopic surgery uses small holes or punctures rather than one large incision. These small incisions result in less postoperative pain and shorter recovery, as compared with an abdominal incision. Women usually return to work within 3 or 4 days after laparoscopy in comparison to 4 to 6 weeks after more extensive surgery.

Many procedures can now be done through a laparoscope:

- Hysterectomy
- Removal of the gallbladder
- Removal of segments of colon

- Assisting vaginal hysterectomy
- Removal of fibroids
- Removal of the fallopian tubes
- Sterilization
- Removal of ovarian cysts

Laser

Laser therapy uses a beam of very intense and focused light to perform surgery. It is used to remove abnormal tissue from the cervix that could be a sign of early cancer. The laser also can remove warts that result from HPV infection. To increase the likelihood of complete cure, a small margin of normal tissue may also be removed. An anesthetic is given before surgery, and recovery is usually very rapid.

Loop Electrosurgical Excision Procedure

For a loop electrosurgical excision procedure, known as LEEP, a high-intensity electrical current passes through a wire used to cut a thin slice of tissue from the cervix. This tissue can be examined under a microscope. In addition to obtaining samples of tissue for diagnosis, LEEP also can be used for treatment by removing abnormal tissue. A local anesthetic is administered before the procedure, and pain medication may be given to ease postoperative discomfort. A minimal discharge is experienced after this procedure.

Ultrasound

In ultrasound, inaudible super-swift sound waves are projected into the body. The reflected echoes are captured to create an image of the internal structures of the body; this is transferred to a black and white image on a monitor screen. From this image the physician or diagnostic expert can tell the size and shape of the ovaries, the uterus, and other pelvic structures. It can determine the age and exact location of the fetus within the uterus. In some situations physical details of a fetus can be identified; it is especially helpful in confirming a possible multiple birth.

CONDITIONS AND DISORDERS IN MEN

When there is a disorder in the reproductive system of men, it can affect several functions, including urination and sexual function.

Benign Prostatic Hyperplasia

The prostate gland continues to grow during most of a man's life. It is common for the prostate gland to become enlarged as a man ages. This growth is called benign prostatic hyperplasia, or BPH. Over half of all men over age 60 and about 90 percent of all men in their 70s and 80s have some symptoms of BPH. Symptoms include a weaker urinary stream and a need to urinate more often, especially at night.

Symptoms are caused by pressure from the prostate growth around the urethra, which obstructs the bladder. The bladder cannot fully empty, leaving urine behind. Eventually this can lead to urinary tract infections, bladder or kidney damage, bladder stones, and incontinence. The cause of BPH is not clear, but is dependent on aging and androgens. Although some of the signs of BPH and prostate cancer are similar, having BPH does not seem to increase the chances of getting prostate cancer.

When BPH causes a partial obstruction of the urethra, certain factors can bring on symptoms. Some over-the-counter cold or allergy medicines can prevent the bladder from allowing urine to pass. Other conditions that can bring on urinary retention include alcohol, cold temperatures, or a long period of immobility.

Treatment may not be required in the early stages. If problems develop, however, medical or surgical treatment may be required. Some medications

STAGES OF PROSTATE CANCER

Stage I	Cancer, confined within the prostate, is not felt or detected but found incidentally after surgery.
Stage II	Cancer, within the prostate, is usually felt on digital rectal exam.
Stage III	Cancer found outside the prostate in adjacent tissues.
Stage IV	Cancer has spread outside the gland and has metastasized to distant tissues.

used to treat BPH shrink the prostate cells or relax the smooth muscle of the prostate. The blood pressure drugs terazosin (Hytrin) and doxazosin can be used to relax smooth muscle in the prostate.

Sometimes, surgery to remove the enlarged part of the prostate is recommended. In most cases, surgery is performed through the urethra with a light-transmitting instrument that has an electrical loop at the end to cut tissue. Surgery can also be performed through an open incision. Most men recover completely within 6 weeks. Sexual function may take a while to return but usually is not affected. After surgery, most men experience retrograde ejaculation, in which they achieve orgasm during sex but the semen travels backwards to the bladder rather than forward out the penis.

Cancer

Prostate Cancer

One of the most common cancers in the United States, close to 200,000 new cases of prostate cancer are diagnosed each year. The prevalence of prostate cancer increases rapidly with age, reaching about 50 percent in men over 70. The cancer incidence is higher in African-American than in white men. In the early stages there are no symptoms.

The cancer is usually discovered by digital rectal examination (DRE), in which a hard lump or growth in the prostate gland can be detected before symptoms develop. Tests are then performed to confirm the diagnosis. In addition to imaging studies, blood tests

to measure a chemical called prostate-specific antigen (PSA) are performed to detect the high levels that
occur in the presence of cancer. Biopsies are done to
obtain a piece of tissue for further study and, if cancer cells are present, the stage of disease is determined (see "Stages of Prostate Cancer").

Treatment can include surgery, radiation therapy, hormone therapy, or a combination of these
treatments. Because prostate cancer cells use the
male hormones to grow, blocking production of
these hormones with gonadotropin androgens and
antiandrogens may control the disease. All of these
treatments have side effects. The chance of complete
cure is good when the disease is detected in its early
stages.

Testicular Cancers

Cancer of the testis is the most common type of cancer in men between the ages of 18 and 35. Two to
three new cases per 100,000 males occur in the
United States each year. White men are four times
more likely than African-American men to develop
testicular cancer. Seminoma, the most common type
of testicular cancer, has a high cure rate when treated early.

Any unusual lump on the testis, or any new
lump, even if it is not painful, should be evaluated by
a physician. When a tumor is found in one testis, surgical removal is required; the remaining testis maintains the body's normal functions. The loss of both
testes results in loss of hormone production, and
testosterone therapy will be necessary to maintain
sexual function.

Cryptorchidism

Cryptorchidism is also known as hidden testis or undescended testis, because the testis has not reached its normal position in the scrotum. A physician can confirm the absence of the testis by feeling the scrotum, and all young boys should be checked early for this condition. The undescended testis must be removed if it cannot be put in the normal scrotal position because it carries increased risk of testicular cancer.

Epididymitis

Infection of the epididymis, the coiled tube that transports sperm to the vas deferens, is caused either by the STDs, including chlamydia and gonorrhea, or by the E. coli bacteria. This condition is easily transmitted and can be very painful. The infecting organism can sometimes be identified in samples of urine. Antibiotics are usually prescribed. Ice packs applied to the scrotum reduce swelling and pain. It is important to distinguish epididymitis from torsion of the testis, which should be treated immediately.

Gynecomastia

Enlargement of the male breasts, know as gynecomastia, can occur on one or both sides. It is usually triggered by an imbalance in the normal ratio of androgen to estrogen in the blood supply—either androgen production is decreased or estrogen levels are increased. Gynecomastia can occur normally in newborns, at adolescence, or with aging. It also can result from several endocrine disorders and some medications; gynecomastia should be evaluated.

Erectile Dysfunction (Impotence)

The inability to have or keep an erection sufficient to permit intercourse or masturbation is called impotence or erectile dysfunction. Nearly every man experiences temporary impotence related to fatigue, stress, or illness. More than 10 million men in the United States are chronically impotent. The problem increases with age; 30 percent of men age 65 have recurrent episodes of impotence.

Many factors can affect the complex interaction of vascular, neurologic, and endocrine systems that allow normal erectile function. Although sexual function and desire may decrease with age, age is not necessarily a cause of impotence. Medication side effects, stress, smoking, and alcoholism can be risk factors. Inadequate testosterone, anxiety, premature ejaculation, and Peyronie's disease are some of the treatable causes of the problem. Diabetes is the most common disease associated with erectile problems.

Treatment requires a medical history and physical examination; this should include an evaluation of testis size, shape, and consistency and palpation of the shaft of the penis. A testosterone level and a nocturnal penile tumescence test can be used to detect whether a man is having an erection at night while he sleeps. If a man is physically able to have an erection, his impotence could be caused by psychological reasons, and he may benefit from counseling.

Some of the methods of treatment include the use of penile or intracavernous injections, vacuum devices, and penile implants. Support groups, changes in lifestyle, or medications can be helpful.

Infertility

Defined as the inability of a couple to conceive after 12 months of unprotected intercourse, infertility is thought to affect 10–15 percent of married couples in the United States. Some of the known causes of male infertility include chromosomal abnormalities, loss of germ cells that produce sperm (which can occur during treatment for cancer), deficient hormones, or physical abnormalities. Infertility can be caused by an inadequate number of sperm, or the sperm may be present but not strong enough to penetrate the egg.

A physician's examination should include palpation of the testes and the epididymis to look for possible obstructions that could prevent sperm from traveling out the penis. A rectal examination should be performed to evaluate the prostate and possible abnormalities of the structures involved in ejaculation. Two or more semen analyses should be done. Additional tests may include evaluation of the hormone testosterone. Treatments are directed at the specific causes identified by the couple's history, the physical exams, and testing.

Peyronie's Disease

In Peyronie's disease a firm plaque or growth occurs on the connective tissue of the penis. This plaque can cause pain during an erection and make vaginal penetration difficult. This growth is not malignant and can go away on its own. If it lasts more than one year, surgery may be helpful.

Premature Ejaculation

Ejaculation that occurs just before or shortly after penetration of the woman is considered premature. Often associated with problems in a relationship, it may also be due to inadequate control over the ejaculatory process and does not have a physical cause.

In the past, treatment included efforts to decrease anxiety by concentrating on nonsexual fantasies, use of cerebral depressants or sedatives, and distractive maneuvers such as compressing the glans of the penis. To decrease penile sensation, anesthetic ointments were applied, condoms were used, and penile movement in the vagina was minimized. Today it is recognized that this is a psychological problem that requires behavioral therapy. Such therapy is usually successful when both partners participate.

Priapism

Priapism is a prolonged, often painful penile erection that lasts for more than 4 to 6 hours. It is not associated with sexual desire. Causes are often unclear but include leukemia or sickle cell anemia. Prolonged erections also can result from the use of drugs and injections into the penis to correct erectile problems. The condition must be treated right away by a urologist to prevent permanent damage to the penis.

Prostatitis

An inflammation of the prostate, prostatitis may arise suddenly or be longlasting or recurring. Symptoms include difficulty urinating; pain in the lower back, muscles, joints, or the area between the scrotum and anus; or painful ejaculation. If untreated, prostatitis can cause abscesses, spread of infection, and urinary retention. Prostatitis is diagnosed by a careful digital rectal examination and urinalysis to identify any bacterial infection. When the condition is caused by bacteria, it is treated with antibiotics; hot baths sometimes provide relief from the symptoms.

Retrograde Ejaculation

In retrograde ejaculation, orgasm occurs, but no ejaculate leaves the penis. This condition usually arises after surgery to remove an enlarged prostate, when the muscles around the bladder neck are removed. Instead of being expelled through the penis, sperm enters the urethra near the opening of the bladder and is flushed out with urine. Although a man may be unable to have children without special assisted techniques, he retains his libido, potency, and ability to have an erection and orgasm.

Testicular Failure

Testicular failure is rare. It is caused by both chromosomal abnormalities as well as damage to the mature testes due to disease or injury. The loss of sex drive typical with this condition often can be restored through a program of androgen replacement. Fertility cannot be restored.

Varicocele

A swelling in the scrotum caused by enlarged veins, varicocele is common in otherwise healthy men. It is caused by problems with the valves located in the veins leading from the testes. The blockage causes blood to back up, resulting in swelling and infertility. When varicocele causes infertility, surgery is necessary.

PROCEDURES FOR MEN

Nocturnal Penile Tumescence Test

Sleep-associated erections can be monitored with the nocturnal penile tumescence test to evaluate impotence. Normal males have three to five erections per night's sleep. Both intrapenile injections and the penile tumescence test may be used in a complete diagnostic evaluation.

Semen Analysis

Semen is collected from a male after 2 or more days of abstinence. Ideally, two or more samples are taken over a 75–90 day period. A normal sperm count is at least 20 million sperm per milliliter. At least 50 percent of the sperm should be moving, with a significant number moving rapidly forward, and at least 50 percent of the sperm should appear normal on microscopic examination. This test should be performed as a part of an infertility evaluation.

Vasectomy

About a half million men in the United States have vasectomies each year. A vasectomy is a disruption of the vas deferens. It often is performed through a small puncture in the scrotum through which the vas (tubes that carry sperm from the testes to the urethra) are tied (see Fig. 1.25). No stitching is required, and the operation takes no more than 10 minutes. Recovery takes about 1 week. A semen analysis must be done to make sure the disruption is complete.

Vasectomies are usually reversible. A vasovasectomy is the rejoining of the two ends of the vas; this procedure has a high success rate, and a pregnancy rate of up to 60 percent can result.

HEALTH CARE PRACTITIONERS

Women can receive care for the reproductive system from any of the following health care professionals:

- Obstetrician-gynecologist: A specialist who has completed 4 years of residency beyond medical school in the field of women's health. This

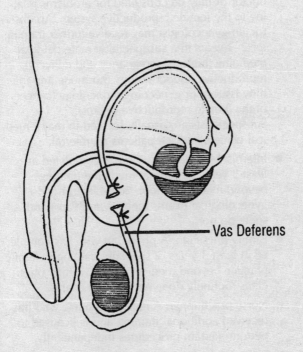

Vas Deferens

Figure 1.25 Vasectomy
Vasectomy, a form of sterilization for men, is a relatively simple procedure that is very effective for the prevention of pregnancy. A small incision is made in the scrotum, and the vas deferens, the tube through which sperm move from the testes to the urethra, is cut and the ends tied off. Reversal of the procedure has a high success rate.

physician may be the woman's primary care doctor or may be consulted for problems relating to the female reproductive system. An obstetrician-gynecologist may receive further training for 2–3 years in a subspecialty: maternal-fetal medicine (high-risk pregnancy and delivery), reproductive endocrinology (hormone and infertility issues), or gynecologic oncology (cancers of the female reproductive organs). Subspecialists are usually located in major medical centers and see patients on referral.

- Internist: A specialist who has completed at least 3 years of internal medicine training beyond medical school. Some internists do gynecological exams (pelvics and Paps) and some do not.

- Family physician: A physician who has completed at least 3 years of specialty training in family practice beyond medical school. Family physicians routinely do gynecological exams.

- Nurse practitioner: A registered nurse who has received additional training and is licensed to perform certain procedures independently.

- Nurse-midwife: A registered nurse who has additional training in providing obstetrical care to women.

For routine examinations, men can see an internal medicine specialist or a family practitioner. A man having a problem with his prostate or infertility may be referred to a urologist for evaluation.

PART II

Pregnancy and Childbirth

Susan Aucott Ballagh, M.D.,
and Barbara Bartlik, M.D.,

Few words trigger a wider range of emotional reactions in women than, "You're pregnant!" Some women are simply ecstatic about their new pregnant state and almost ready to name the baby they won't meet for many months. Other women are frightened and uncertain about their condition and not quite ready for the upheaval a child can bring. Yet no matter how a woman reacts psychologically, ignorance is never bliss when it comes to pregnancy and childbirth. The more information a woman has about this special time, the better equipped she is to meet its challenges.

In almost no other stage of life are there so many changes and challenges in such a brief time. For most women, pregnancy lasts approximately 40 weeks or 280 days, counting from the first day of the last menstrual period (see "How to Calculate Your Due Date"). Compared to the number of years in a healthy woman's life, 280 days isn't a very long time.

During pregnancy, a woman is really two people at once; she's eating, breathing, and being responsible for her own health as well as that of her baby. It is an exciting time, but one that can be filled with conflicting emotions. Most pregnant women face uncertainties about pregnancy and some anxiety about what the future holds. You can be better prepared if you plan for your pregnancy and what it will entail, understand the changes that are taking place and learn ways to cope with them, and become actively involved in your prenatal care.

HOW TO CALCULATE YOUR DUE DATE

To calculate your due date...

- Count 280 days from the first day of your last period.

or

- Count back three months from the first day of the last menstrual period and add seven days.

   This is only a guide. Very few women actually deliver their babies on this expected day of arrival.

PRECONCEPTIONAL CARE

A woman who is planning to become pregnant may benefit from preconceptional care (see "Components of Preconceptional Care"). Such care is usually provided by an obstetrician-gynecologist. It is designed to identify risks or problems before pregnancy, provide information about any special needs a woman may have to prepare for pregnancy, and make sure a woman is as healthy as possible before she becomes pregnant.

   Preconceptional care is important because the organs of the fetus (unborn baby) begin to form as early as day 17 of the pregnancy. The fetus may be exposed to health risks before a woman or her doctor even know she is pregnant. Preconceptional care is especially important for women who have certain

COMPONENTS OF PRECONCEPTIONAL CARE

The following items may be covered during a preconceptional visit:

- Assessment of medical, reproductive, and family history; nutritional status; drug exposures
- Possible effects of pregnancy on existing medical conditions
- Genetic concerns
- Immunization against infections
- Laboratory tests
- Nutritional counseling
- Discussion of social, financial, and psychological issues and concerns

medical conditions, such as hypertension and diabetes, which can affect the health of the fetus if they are not under control before pregnancy. Multivitamins containing at least 400 micrograms of folic acid reduce fetal malformations.

IN THE BEGINNING

Every month, at about day 14 of a 28-day menstrual cycle, one of a woman's ovaries releases an egg; this is called ovulation. If a man's sperm penetrates the egg, fertilization takes place. The sperm fuses with the egg and forms a single cell. This cell begins to divide and travel down the fallopian tube. It reaches the uterus about the fourth day after fertilization. Now a cluster of about 100 fluid-filled cells, the egg floats until day five to eight when it becomes implanted in the lining of the uterus (endometrium).

The outer cells start to spread into the lining to form a blood supply right next to the mother's blood system, called the placenta. The placenta is actually a life-support system because it provides the fetus with food and oxygen and takes away waste products. The placenta also produces human chorionic gonadotropin (hCG), the hormone which signals the beginning of a new life. This hormone maintains the corpus luteum in the ovary which provides progesterone to the growing fetus.

The placenta connects the mother and the fetus. The umbilical cord links the fetus to the placenta. The fetus floats in a sac of amniotic fluid throughout pregnancy. This fluid regulates the unborn baby's temperature and acts as a shock absorber, protecting the fetus from injury.

CONFIRMING PREGNANCY

Even though every woman is different, in the first weeks after conception, some early signs of pregnancy occur. Some of these symptoms may disappear completely after the end of the first three months of pregnancy.

- Missing a period (it is possible to be pregnant and still bleed around the time a period would normally occur)
- Tender breasts

- Nausea and vomiting, often (but not always) in the mornings
- Fatigue
- Need to urinate frequently
- Aching or heaviness in the pelvic area

Kits for home pregnancy testing are available in most pharmacies. All rely on a chemical that, when combined with your urine in a little test tube, changes colors in the presence of hCG. Follow the directions of home kits carefully. Though up to 98 percent correct, if the test is performed too early, before hCG levels have risen, the results can be falsely negative. The test should be done at least 10–14 days after a period has been missed. It may be necessary to repeat the test.

About two weeks after a missed period, a doctor, nurse-midwife, or health care practitioner can confirm the pregnancy by testing a sample of blood or urine and examining the pelvic organs to detect changes that occur during pregnancy. Make plans then to begin a prenatal care program.

PROFESSIONAL SUPPORT

Care during pregnancy and birth can be provided by an obstetrician, a family practitioner, or a nurse-midwife. Ideally, a health professional should be selected before pregnancy. If you don't already have a doctor or nurse-midwife in whom you have confidence and trust, start searching for one right away. Recommendations can be made by family and friends, as well as the local medical society.

The American College of Obstetricians and Gynecologists can provide a list of specialists in the area. Write to their resource center at 409 Twelfth Street SW, Washington, DC 20024. To find a nurse-midwife, contact the American College of Nurse-Midwives, 1522 K Street NW, Washington, DC 20005, and send a self-addressed, stamped envelope.

To check the credentials of any physician in a specialty, phone the American Board of Medical Specialists' toll-free number, 800-776-2378. Specialists like obstetrician-gynecologists have 4 years of extra training beyond medical school and have passed certifying exams in their area of expertise. This information is available via the hotline.

Following are some points to consider when selecting a health care provider:

- In what hospital does the doctor or midwife have privileges to practice? Is the location convenient?

- How much will care cost and what does the fee include? What type of insurance is accepted? What does it cover?

- What type of birthing rooms are available? Are there choices regarding the setting?

- What are the health professionals' policies regarding episiotomies (a cut made between the vagina and the anus near the end of labor to help the baby's head pass through)? What options are available for pain relief?

- Can special care be provided for any complications that you may have?

- Is there a special neonatal unit or, if not, where will any baby who needs extra help be transferred?

The setting for giving birth should also be considered. Some hospitals have equipped labor rooms, called birthing rooms, with special beds and technical supports so labor and delivery can take place in one room, instead of moving the woman to a delivery room for birth. An alternative birthing center is a facility separate from the hospital where women give birth. Some have a relationship with a hospital so facilities can be shared and others do not. Most have comfortable settings for childbirth.

An interview with a provider being considered may be useful to answer these questions or any others that arise. Once a provider has been selected, prenatal care (a program of care for a pregnant woman before the birth of her baby) should begin.

PRENATAL CARE

With an uncomplicated pregnancy, visits to the doctor or nurse-midwife usually take place once a month during the initial six months and then every two or three weeks thereafter. The first visit is longer than the others and includes a health history, a thorough physical examination (including blood pressure, height and weight measurements), and tests. The internal reproductive organs are examined to check for changes in the cervix and the size of the uterus. Tests performed at the first visit include:

- Blood tests to check for the blood type, Rh factor, anemia, immunity to rubella (German measles), hepatitis B virus, and some sexually transmitted diseases (STDs).

- Urine tests to give information about sugar (which might be a sign of diabetes), protein (signaling possible kidney changes), and signs of infection.

- A Pap test to detect changes in the cervix that could be an early sign of cancer.

Some tests may be repeated at subsequent visits. Other tests may be offered based on risk factors (see "Prenatal Tests"). These tests include those to detect genetic disorders, some of which are offered routinely and some of which are recommended for special circumstances.

After the first visit, most visits can be brief. Each one, however, is a good opportunity to ask questions and gather information on prenatal classes (see "Childbirth Preparation"). Each prenatal visit includes:

- Sampling urine to check for sugar and protein

- Measuring blood pressure to see if levels are normal

- Assessing weight to be sure you are gaining enough

- Listening to the heartbeat of the fetus (after 12 weeks)

- Checking the size and position of the uterus and fetus

At each prenatal visit you should discuss with your doctor any changes that may have occurred since the last visit. Also, share any concerns you have and discuss how you should modify your lifestyle to promote a healthy pregnancy.

Prenatal Tests

The following prenatal tests may be offered to certain women based on their patient histories and the results of routine tests:

Maternal Serum Screening

Certain tests can be performed on the mother's blood to detect substances from the fetus that could signal a birth defect. These tests are usually offered to all women at about 15–18 weeks of pregnancy. One of the substances tested is alpha-fetoprotein (AFP). High levels could be a sign of a neural tube defect, which results when the brain or spinal cord do not develop properly. Low levels could be a sign of Down syndrome. In some cases, the AFP test is combined with other tests to give more accurate results. Abnormal results require further testing, but most babies tested turn out to be normal.

Ultrasound

Ultrasound creates a picture of the fetus by beaming sound waves into the body and reflecting them on a screen. It is done if there is a question about the status or age of the fetus or to confirm the results of other tests. It can be done at various times during pregnancy, depending on the reason. A thin layer of jelly is rubbed on the mother's belly, and a handheld instrument, called a transducer, is passed over it. Ultrasound determines whether the baby is growing normally, positioning in the womb, abnormalities, or if there is more than one fetus.

Amniocentesis

For an amniocentesis test, the fetal cells in the amniotic fluid are analyzed for signs of birth defects. This test is performed between the 14th and 18th week of pregnancy. A small amount of fluid is removed with a needle from the sac surrounding the baby. The test is recommended for women 35 or older at the time of delivery because they have a higher risk of having a baby with Down syndrome. In addition, it is given to women who have had a previous child with a birth defect, or who have a family or personal history that places them at risk for an inherited disease. Amniocentesis also may follow abnormal serum tests. There is a small risk of miscarriage with the test. (See Fig. 2.1)

Chorionic Villus Sampling (CVS)
A sample of chorionic villi, the fetal blood vessels that form part of the placenta, is removed and analyzed for

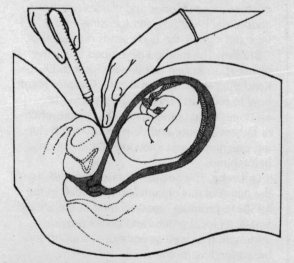

Figure 2.1   Amniocentesis
A needle is inserted into the uterus to obtain a sample of the amniotic fluid. This fluid contains cells of the fetus that can be studied to detect disorders.

CHILDBIRTH PREPARATION

Childbirth preparation can include lectures, exercise instructions, and tours of maternity/obstetrics departments. They may combine several theories of how to manage labor. There are various techniques. Most courses can be taken in a hospital or privately.

Lamaze. Named after a French doctor, Fernand Lamaze, these classes stress breathing exercises for each stage of labor, along with relaxation techniques. Also emphasized is the need to focus on something almost hypnotically to take your mind off your labor pains.

Dick-Read. Grantly Dick-Read is a British doctor whose theories and classes emphasize abdominal breathing and focusing on the feelings and signals the body sends during labor.

Bradley. The method developed by Denver obstetrician Robert Bradley is closer to Dick-Read than to Lamaze in theory. Couples learn how to relax and breathe deeply. Emphasis is on doing what comes naturally, the presence of fathers at labor and delivery, nutrition during pregnancy, and knowing all the options beforehand.

La Leche. The Spanish phrase, *the milk,* is the name of this organization founded in the 1950s to promote breast-feeding in the United States. Its local groups and books provide information as well as emotional support for breast-feeding mothers.

this test. It is done at 10–12 weeks of pregnancy. CVS is offered for chromosomal screening. This test may not be available in all areas, and there is a slight risk of miscarriage. Some women choose this test over amniocentesis because the results are available earlier.

Fetal Monitoring

Two forms of monitoring may be done during pregnancy, usually in the last 10 weeks, to check the well-being of the fetus. One is the nonstress test, which measures the fetal heartrate in response to its own movements. The other is the contraction stress test that measures how the fetal heart rate responds to the stress of a uterine contraction. For both tests, a device is strapped to the mother's abdomen and the results are recorded on a tracing. For the contraction stress test, mild uterine contractions are induced with a drug called oxytocin.

GROWTH AND DEVELOPMENT

When the fertilized egg becomes implanted in the uterus it begins to divide and grow. For the first 8 weeks of pregnancy, the egg is called an embryo. After that, it is called a fetus, which literally means "young one."

First Month (See Fig. 2.2)

- Inside a fluid-filled sac, the embryo has a simple brain, spine, and central nervous system.
- The circulatory system as well as the start of a digestive system have begun to form.

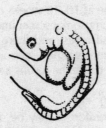

Figure 2.2 Five-Six Weeks

Second Month (See Fig. 2.3)

- The heart begins to beat in the tiny body, somewhere between the size of an apple seed and a green grape (1/2 inch).
- Spots appear where eyes will form and a face is almost recognizable.
- Arms and legs are present as little buds growing longer each day.
- An outline of the nervous system is present and major internal organs appear in a simple form.

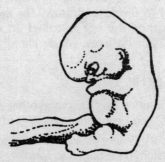

Figure 2.3 Seven-Eight Weeks

Third Month (See Fig. 2.4)

- The fetus is the size of a tennis ball, about 2¹/₂ inches long and weighs about one-twentieth of a pound (14 grams).
- Fingers and toes are now in place.
- Ears, as well as earlobes, are developed.
- Eyelids close over the eyes and the muscles of the face are mature enough to allow movement of the face and lips.
- Vocal cords are complete.

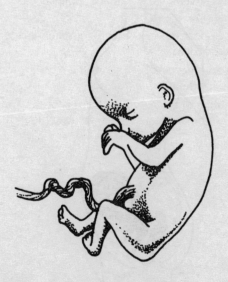

Figure 2.4   Twelve Weeks

Fourth Month (See Fig. 2.5)

■ The fetus is fully formed and approximately 5 inches long, weighing about 4 ounces (110 grams). Using the placenta as a lifeline, the fetus now takes in lots of oxygen, food, and water.

■ The fetus can suck a thumb.

■ Eyebrows and eyelashes are growing.

■ The fetal heart beats twice as fast as the mother's and can be heard with a special listening device (doppler ultrasound).

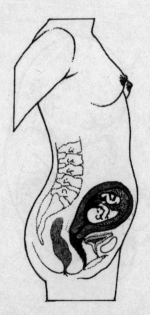

Figure 2.5 Four Months

Fifth Month (See Fig. 2.6)

- An old-fashioned term referring to fetal movement is *quickening*, generally thought to mean "feeling life." It feels like a faint flutter, a slight tickling sensation, or perhaps even bubbles.

- The unborn baby has hair on the head and is developing teeth. It is 6½ inches long and weighs ¾ of a pound (350 grams).

- A white, greasy substance called vernix covers the skin and protects it.

- Fine hair called lanugo covers the fetus.

- Facial features are wrinkled and shriveled.

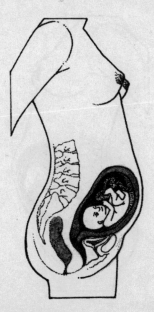

Figure 2.6   Five Months

Sixth Month (See Fig. 2.7)

- The fetus tries out leg and arm muscles often and can have periods of frenzied activity, kicking, punching, and even turning somersaults.

- Ten inches long and about 2 pounds (1000 grams), the fetus can cough, hiccup, and respond to sudden noises.

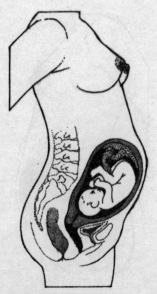

Figure 2.7 Six Months

Seventh Month (See Fig. 2.8)

- The baby's eyes have opened and taste buds are forming. The part of the brain that controls intelligence and temperament is developing. Soon evidence of a personality appears.

- The baby's skin is wrinkled but an underlayering of fat is slowly building. Lungs are better developed, but a substance called surfactant is still missing. Surfactant keeps newborn lungs from collapsing between each breath.

- The baby is now 12 inches long and weighs about 3 1/2 pounds (1700 grams).

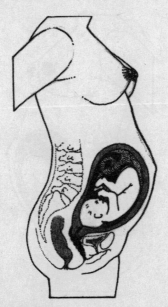

Figure 2.8 Seven Months

Eighth Month (See Fig. 2.9)

- The fetus is probably in the position in which most babies are born: head down, pushing on the pubic area, especially if this is a first birth. This is the cephalic position.

- Bones harden, but the head bones remain soft and flexible for delivery.

- The baby measures about 16 inches and weighs about 5½ pounds (2500 grams).

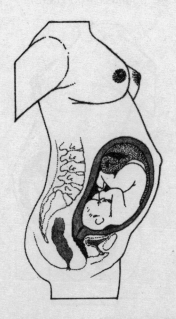

Figure 2.9   Eight Months

Ninth Month (See Fig. 2.10)

- The baby gains about an ounce a day now. If it's a boy, the testicles have descended.

- Nails have grown to cover fingers and toes.

- The lanugo hair and most of the vernix disappear.

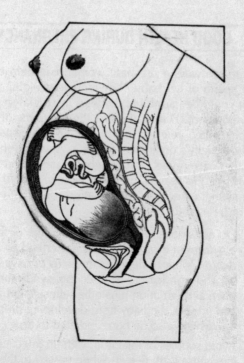

Figure 2.10   Nine Months
The fetus drops into the birth position as your due date nears.

Full Term

- A substance called meconium is now present in the baby's intestines. This becomes the first bowel movement after birth.

- At term (40 weeks) the average baby is about 20 inches long and weighs 7½ pounds (normal range is 6–9 pounds).

GOOD HEALTH DURING PREGNANCY

There are ways a pregnant woman can help ensure the health of her baby. They include avoiding things that could be harmful to the fetus in crucial stages of development. During the first three months of pregnancy, often referred to as the first trimester, the unborn baby's organs are forming. Anything that the mother eats, drinks, and breathes is passed on to the fetus. For this reason, pregnant women should avoid things that can cause complications during pregnancy or be harmful to the fetus:

- Do not smoke tobacco, drink alcohol, or take any form of drug unless it is prescribed by a doctor. Tobacco deprives the fetus of oxygen. Alcohol can lead to fetal alcohol syndrome (mental retardation plus other effects). Drugs can prevent the baby from developing properly. Babies can also be born addicted to drugs.

- Avoid sources of infection. Certain infections can cause birth defects when passed to the fetus during pregnancy or birth. They include toxo-

WHERE DOES THE WEIGHT GO?

A woman of average weight should gain about 30 pounds during her pregnancy. Here is how it's distributed:

- 38% baby
- 22% blood and fluid
- 20% womb, breasts, buttocks, legs
- 11% amniotic fluid
- 9% placenta

plasmosis, an infection caused by a parasite in cat feces and raw meat, rubella (if a woman is not immune), syphilis, hepatitis B, and other sexually transmitted diseases.

- Avoid hazards in the workplace. They include chemicals, gas, dust, fumes, or radiation. Also, avoid lifting heavy loads or standing all day.
- Avoid household hazards such as cleaning products, fumes, or paints.
- Avoid high body temperature whether due to illness, baths, saunas, or hot tubs.

To maintain your health and that of your baby eat right to support the growth of the fetus, exercise to strengthen muscles and ease discomforts, and get enough sleep.

A woman of normal weight should gain approximately 30 pounds during pregnancy (see "Where Does the Weight Go?"). Women who are overweight should gain less. Teenagers and women who are underweight or carrying twins should gain more. Pregnancy is not a time to try to lose weight. You need about 2,400 calories per day during pregnancy (about 300 calories more than a nonpregnant woman). You also need extra iron, folic acid, and calcium to provide nutrients for the fetus.

Exercise can help a pregnant woman prepare for birth and make her more comfortable during pregnancy. Although this is not the time to take up a hard new sport, if you had been exercising before becoming pregnant, you could continue to do so. Your exercise program may need to be modified because of some of the changes that take place during pregnancy. Your center of gravity, and thus your balance, changes with the added weight, and the hormones of pregnancy cause joints to become more flexible and subject to injury. When exercising, avoid becoming overheated or very tired, drink lots of water, and move more slowly and without jarring motions. Moderate exercise, such as swimming and walking, are good choices; exercises to strengthen back muscles can relieve back pain. However, exercise while lying on the back reduces blood flow to the fetus and is best avoided.

CHANGES DURING PREGNANCY

A woman goes through many emotional and physical changes during her pregnancy. Each woman is different, however, and these changes don't occur in all women or at the same times. Many of these changes are related to the pressure exerted on various parts of the body as the fetus grows.

Emotions

Pregnancy is a turning point in a woman's life. As with other phases of transition, psychological issues may resurface during this time. Often the woman revisits her own childhood experience and recalls the way in which she was raised.

The first three months of pregnancy are a time of adjusting to, or coming to terms with, the pregnancy. The middle of pregnancy is a relatively quiet time, during which the woman begins the process of bonding with the baby. Knowing the sex of the child in advance, which is available through some prenatal tests, may promote bonding. The pregnant woman may withdraw from outside activities and focus on her relationship with the baby's father and her home life. These feelings continue to grow into the last part of pregnancy. There may be increased anxiety and fear of problems about the delivery at this time.

Sexuality

Sexuality changes during pregnancy. For some women, the increased levels of hormones enhance their desire for sex during pregnancy. For others, sexual functioning increases at certain phases and decreases at others. A number of factors may interfere with sexual functioning. They include nausea, physical discomfort, fear of harming the fetus, feeling less desirable with increased weight, and bodily changes. Changes in the partner's responsiveness are also a factor. Some men draw closer to their partner during pregnancy and the postpartum period, but others may go through psychological changes, causing them to withdraw from the relationship. The woman's new maternal role, and her new physical appearance, may bring out unresolved conflicts in her partner.

Some couples are concerned that having sex during pregnancy can harm the fetus. In most cases it will not because the fetus is cushioned by the sac of amniotic fluid. A couple may find it more comfortable to try different positions that don't place pressure on a woman's abdomen. If there is a complication or concern, the doctor or nurse-midwife may suggest that the couple abstain from sex.

Sleeping Problems

Early pregnancy is often associated with prolonged sleep and fatigue. Sleep disturbance is also noted during pregnancy. For some women it may be the first symptom of pregnancy. It is quite common for women to have difficulty falling asleep or staying asleep at any given time during the pregnancy. Sleep may be particularly disturbed as term approaches. Some women dream vividly. Sleeping medications are best avoided because they could harm the fetus, especially during early pregnancy. Warm baths, relaxation exercises, and lying on one side propped by a pillow may help. (See Fig. 2.11)

Backache

As they get ready for the strain of delivery, joints and ligaments in your body relax. The result could be a backache. Exercises can help promote good posture and relieve aching muscles. To avoid back injury, avoid lifting whenever possible. If you must lift, bend from the knees, keeping the back straight. Do not lie flat on your back because the supine position can make it hard to breathe, and reduce blood flow to the baby.

Breast Changes

One of the first signs of pregnancy is tender breasts. The breasts continue to grow and change throughout pregnancy to prepare for breast-feeding. The nipples and surrounding skin might become darker, and the nipples and veins become more prominent. A woman's bra size may increase to twice the original size during pregnancy. Wear a comfortable cotton bra with wide shoulder straps and deep bands under the cups. Late in pregnancy, a woman may notice a yellow, watery fluid leaking from her nipples. This is called colostrum, and it nourishes the baby in the first days of life. It is rich in protective substances, called antibodies, which fight infection.

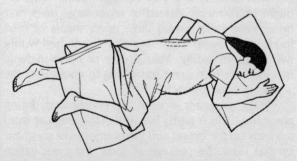

Figure 2.11   It may be more comfortable to sleep on one side with one leg propped up on a pillow.

Breathing Problems

The pressure of the uterus on the bottom of the rib cage can cause a feeling of shortness of breath. The lungs do not have room enough to expand and take in enough air. In late pregnancy just before birth, the fetus drops and this often relieves that feeling.

Gastrointestinal Problems

Most women have morning sickness—nausea and vomiting—during the first three months of pregnancy. It usually, but not always, goes away in the middle of pregnancy. The condition is worse when the stomach is empty. Eating a number of small meals a day may help.

Heartburn, or indigestion, has nothing to do with the heart. It is caused by acids from the stomach that cause a burning sensation in the throat and chest. Changes in the hormone levels during pregnancy slow digestion and relax the muscles that keep the stomach acids where they belong. Again, more frequent small meals instead of fewer large ones may bring some relief. Avoid large, spicy meals or fried foods. Also, avoid exercising or going to bed within two hours of eating. Your doctor or nurse-midwife may be able to suggest something to counteract the acidity in your stomach.

Many pregnant women are constipated during pregnancy. This is partly because of the pressure from the fetus on the bowel and the hormones of pregnancy that slow the passage of food. Exercise, eating foods high in fiber, and drinking fluids can help relieve constipation.

Hemorrhoids are enlarged or weakened veins near the anus. The baby's head creates pressure on these veins, causing them to swell during pregnancy. Straining during bowel movements makes the situation worse, causing itching, soreness, and perhaps even bleeding. Increasing fiber and fluid intake, using products for treating hemorrhoids and relieving constipation may help. You should of course consult your doctor before taking any medication.

Skin Changes

A dark line, called the linea nigra, may appear down the center of the stretched stomach, and the skin may itch. Skin on the abdomen and breasts must expand, often causing streaks called stretch marks. There is no way to prevent these marks; many lighten after birth. In some women, the hormones produced during pregnancy cause a brown mask on the face called chloasma that often fades after birth when hormones return to normal.

Varicose Veins

Swollen and painful veins, called varicose veins, often occur in the calves, thighs, and the vagina. They are made worse by poor circulation in the legs, especially during long periods of standing. Special support stockings can be worn to relieve aching, sore legs. Also helpful is lying on your side, with legs elevated, as is floating in water. While standing, move around as much as possible, lifting heels or toes to promote circulation.

Swelling

Most women have some degree of swelling in the legs or the hands during pregnancy. The face also may puff up because of the body's tendency to retain fluid. Although extreme swelling can be a sign that the kidneys are not working properly, some swelling is normal. Resting on your side with the feet elevated can help. In the third trimester, floating in water can help relieve swelling.

Other Changes

- Swollen gums that bleed more easily
- Muscle and leg cramps
- Numbness and tingling in the extremities
- Thicker hair growth
- Need to urinate more often (remember, sudden increases may signal infection)

SPECIAL CONSIDERATIONS

Some pregnancies require special care. In some cases this is known in advance. In others, warning signs occur during the course of pregnancy and are detected during prenatal care. Any warning signs should be reported to the clinician right away (see "Warning Signs").

Miscarriage

Miscarriage, also called spontaneous abortion, is the loss of a pregnancy before the fetus can live on its own. It occurs in about 15 percent of pregnancies, usually in early pregnancy. Most miscarriages occur

---

WARNING SIGNS

Any of the following symptoms could be a sign of a problem and require immediate medical attention:

- Vaginal bleeding can be a sign of a miscarriage or a problem with the placenta.

- Vaginal discharge—either a change in the type or an increase in the amount—could be a sign of preterm labor or infection.

- Cramps and back pain could signal miscarriage or preterm birth.

- Swelling, headache, blurred vision occur with high blood pressure in pregnancy.

- Severe, sharp abdominal pain should be evaluated if it doesn't improve with position changes.

- Fever or chills may be symptoms of infection.

- Fluid discharge from your vagina may signal that the amniotic sac has ruptured and labor may begin soon.

- Decreased fetal movement for 12 hours after week 28 could mean the unborn baby is in trouble.

in the first trimester, before 12 weeks. After week 16, the chance of having a miscarriage is low. The risk of miscarriage increases with age.

Miscarriage usually cannot be prevented and often occurs because the pregnancy is not normal. A miscarriage doesn't mean that a woman can't have children in the future. There is no proof that stress or physical or sexual activity causes miscarriage.

An early warning may be vaginal spotting. Other signs of a miscarriage are pain in the lower back, cramps in the lower abdomen, and heavy bleeding with clots. After a miscarriage, a procedure called dilation and curettage (D&C) may be necessary to open and clean the uterus. Loss of a pregnancy through miscarriage is traumatic, emotionally as well as physically. Discuss any concerns about current or future pregnancies with your health care professional. Special tests, procedures, or medicine may be needed if a woman experiences a loss after 12 weeks or if she loses several pregnancies in a row.

Preterm Labor

If labor begins before the 37th week of pregnancy, the baby may be born early. Often, labor can be stopped to allow the fetus more time in the uterus, where it has the best chance of growing and developing normally. Treatments to stop labor include bed rest, fluids given intravenously, and special agents to relax the uterus. The goal is to prolong the pregnancy until the fetus is fully developed. Today, even very early preterm infants can survive in neonatal intensive care units and drugs are available to help their lungs function better.

Problems with the Placenta

In late pregnancy, bleeding can be a sign of problems with the placenta. The placenta may pull away from the wall of the uterus (placental abruption), or it may cover the cervix (placenta previa). Both of these conditions can interfere with the oxygen supply of the fetus and require medical attention. These conditions may be best treated with a cesarean section.

Medical Conditions

High blood pressure and diabetes can develop during pregnancy in women who did not previously have these conditions. They often go away after delivery, although they can recur. These conditions can become worse in women who had them before they became pregnant. In either case, they require treatment.

High blood pressure, coupled with protein in the urine and swelling, is called preeclampsia. Symptoms include headaches, swelling of the hands and face, dizziness, blurred vision, sudden or uneven weight gain, and stomach pain. It can cause seizures and preterm birth and should be treated right away.

Diabetes that occurs during pregnancy is called gestational diabetes. Women with this condition have too much sugar in their blood because the hormones of pregnancy alter the way in which the body processes sugar. When blood sugar is high, the baby may become too large to pass through the mother's birth canal. Diabetes may be controlled through diet, exercise, or insulin (the hormone that processes sugar in the blood). Pills to control glucose are best avoided in pregnancy.

Rh Disease

Antigens are proteins found on the surfaces of blood cells that cause an immune response. One type of antigen is the Rh factor. If the mother's blood lacks the Rh antigen (Rh negative) and the father's blood contains it, the fetus can get the antigen from the father and be Rh positive.

The blood cells from an Rh positive baby can cause an Rh negative mother to produce anti-Rh antibodies as if she were allergic to the fetus. This is called sensitization. Her antibodies cross the placenta, causing anemia or Rh disease. This disease can be prevented by giving the mother a blood product called Rh immunoglobulin (RhIG). This product should be given at any time fetal blood might mix with mother's blood—for example, after an abortion, amniocentesis or chorionic villus testing—to keep antibodies from forming. Once antibodies are formed, they do not go away. RhIG is recommended at 28 weeks of pregnancy for women who are Rh-negative and not sensitized, unless the baby's father is also Rh negative. If her baby has Rh-positive blood, she should be given another dose shortly after she gives birth.

LABOR AND BIRTH

No two women experience exactly the same sensations during labor. Nor are all labors and the accompanying contractions the same length of time. Even expectant mothers who already have children can't be too sure about what might happen. Each baby is different, just as each birth experience holds surprises. What's important is that you understand the various stages of labor and delivery and, if possible, have someone available for support.

Stages of Labor

There are two main parts of the uterus: the upper part is muscular and can expand—its very top part is called the fundus—and at the bottom of the uterus the opening or cervix. In active childbirth, both parts of the uterus work together, contracting and pushing the baby down until the cervix dilates, or opens. The cervix is closed by a ring of muscles that gradually opens and thins (or effaces) during labor. (See Fig. 2.12)

A woman's body gradually prepares for labor and delivery during the last weeks of pregnancy. In those last weeks, the uterus may start to cramp. The cramps become stronger as the due date approaches. These are called Braxton-Hicks contractions or false labor. These contractions differ from true labor in a number of ways (see "True versus False Labor").

About 24 hours before active labor begins, the tiny mucus plug that has guarded the entrance to the cervix may break loose. This is called *bloody show* because blood could be present in the mucus.

Once contractions begin, start timing how long each one lasts and how long it is from the start of one to the start of the next and note the times. If the contractions last 30–70 seconds, if they occur regularly, and if they don't go away with movement, it's probably the real thing. Contact your clinician. A first labor lasts on average 12–14 hours. Labor may be shorter for subsequent births.

There are three stages of labor. Changes take place in each stage, although they vary from one woman to another.

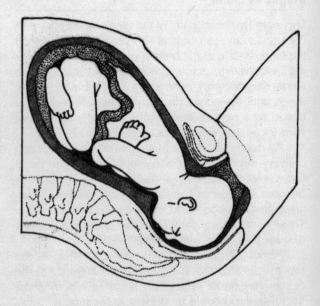

Figure 2.12   Second Stage of Labor.
Contractions of the uterus push the baby through the fully opened cervix.

TRUE VERSUS FALSE LABOR

In true labor, contractions are

- Regular and get closer together
- Continuous in spite of movement
- Usually felt in the back and move to the front
- Increasing steadily in strength

In false labor, contractions are

- Irregular and do not get closer
- Stopped with movement or a change in position
- Often felt in the abdomen
- Weak and do not get stronger

First Stage

The first stage of labor begins when the cervix starts to open and ends when it is fully open. It occurs in three parts: early, active, and transition. In the hospital or clinic, an exam is done to see how labor is progressing.

- *Early Phase.* Contractions are usually mild, lasting 60–90 seconds and occurring every 15–20 minutes. They gradually become more regular and occur less than 5 minutes apart.
- *Active Phase.* Contractions are much stronger, lasting for about 45 seconds and occurring every 3 minutes. Tensing or pushing during this phase is discouraged.

■ *Transition.* Transition is the most difficult stage of labor. The cervix is fully dilated, and contractions occur 2–3 minutes apart and last about 60 seconds. A wave of nausea is commonly noted, which passes rapidly.

Second Stage

The cervix is fully dilated and the baby is ready to be pushed out. Though it's tough physical work—especially in a long labor—it may be more rewarding and contractions may seem less intense. This stage includes the birth of the baby.

■ The second stage may last 2 hours or longer

■ Contractions slow to 2–5 minutes apart and last 60–90 seconds.

■ Pushing should only be done during contractions, with resting and deep breathing between contractions.

■ Maternal coordination and effort can speed delivery.

As the baby's head moves closer to the vaginal opening, it bulges and bumps against the pelvic floor with each contraction. In between contractions, the head may slip back inside. This back and forth motion is normal.

Pushing should stop as soon as the head crowns or becomes visible, to prevent tearing of your skin. At this point an episiotomy, or surgical cut, may be performed to widen the opening. (See Fig. 2.13) You may notice a stinging sensation or numbness as the baby is born because the skin has stretched so much.

In a normal birth, the baby's head slips out first,

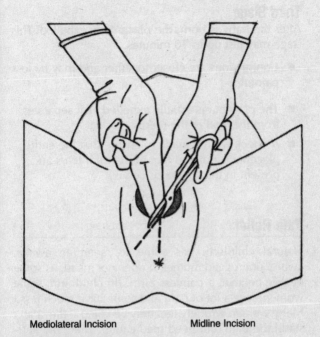

Mediolateral Incision   Midline Incision

Figure 2.13 Episiotomy.
The skin in the perineum (area between the vulva and the rectum)
may be cut just before birth to keep it from tearing. Either a mediolateral or midline incision may be used. The cut is closed with
stitches after birth.

face down. The attendant checks to make sure the
umbilical cord is not wrapped around the neck. The
head turns so one side is lined up with the shoulders.
Fluid or mucus may need to be sucked from the
baby's mouth and nose. With the next contractions,
the body slides out.

Third Stage

After the baby is born, the placenta is expelled. This stage may last up to 30 minutes.

- Contractions are closer together and may be less painful.

- The placenta is usually expelled as it separates from the wall of the uterus.

- A check will be made to ensure that the entire placenta is out and that no harmful tears are present in the vagina or cervix.

Pain Relief

Natural childbirth has come to mean an awake, aware, undrugged mother. It does *not* mean, as some people believe, a painless birth. (In childbirth, some women have a lot of pain and some have much less.) Many women wrongly feel they've failed if they can't stand the pain and need medication. There are various options available, and you need not hesitate to take advantage of them.

Epidural Block

Epidural anesthesia relieves pain during labor, by numbing the area from the waist down. It takes about 10 minutes for an anesthesiologist to administer the medication through a tube inserted between the vertebrae of the backbone. (See Fig. 2.14) An intravenous line is inserted so fluids and medication can be given to prevent blood pressure changes. Complications can include a drop in the mother's blood pressure, which may affect the baby's heartbeat, and a headache, relieved by lying down for a few days after the birth.

Spinal Block
Similar to an epidural, a spinal block is injected into the spinal fluid sac and anesthetizes the body from the waist down. (See Fig. 2.14) Pain relief lasts about 1–2 hours. The injection is given only once during labor, so it is best suited for pain relief during delivery. Complications are similar to those of epidural block.

Pudendal Block
An injection is given shortly before delivery to block pain in the vagina and rectum as the baby is born. It is one of the safest forms of anesthesia.

General Anesthetic
Medications that produce loss of consciousness can be used during cesarean delivery if there is an emergency. One complication is aspiration, when food from a woman's stomach enters the windpipe and lungs, causing injury. This is why a woman should not eat once active labor has begun.

Pain Medications
Drugs can be injected into a muscle or vein to relieve pain. These drugs can have side effects and slow the baby's reflexes and breathing. They usually are given in small doses and avoided just before delivery.

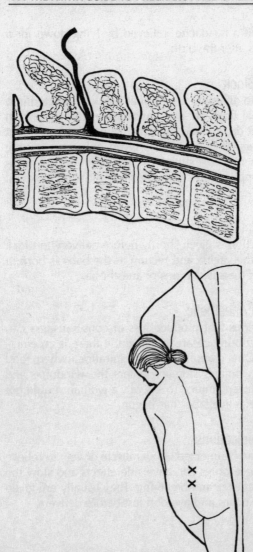

Figure 2.14 Spinal and Epidural Block Anesthesia.
Both spinal and epidural anesthesia are given by an injection in the lower back (A). Spinal anesthesia is injected into the fluid surrounding the spinal cord. Epidural anesthesia is injected into the space outside the spinal cord covering (B).

Monitoring the Fetus

During labor, the status of the baby is monitored by listening to its heartbeat. This process, called auscultation, is done with a special stethoscope, or an electronic fetal monitor, a machine which records the heartbeat.

Auscultation

The heartbeat is monitored by a doctor or nurse, who listens to it at regular intervals. Usually the heartbeat is checked and recorded after a contraction. The frequency of monitoring depends on the stage of labor.

Electronic Fetal Monitoring (EFM)

The two kinds of EFM are external and internal. With external monitoring, an instrument using sound waves (doppler ultrasound) is attached to the mother's abdomen to record the heart rate of the fetus. With internal monitoring, a small device called an electrode is attached to the scalp of the fetus. Sometimes a tube called a catheter is inserted into the uterus to measure uterine contractions. External and internal monitoring techniques may be used together. Both techniques are done to assess whether the fetus is getting enough oxygen and prevent stress. With internal monitoring, the amniotic sac is broken for the device to be inserted in the uterus.

Assisted Delivery

Sometimes the mother needs a helping hand. If she is having trouble during labor, or if labor is delayed, the doctor may use certain tools designed to help speed delivery.

Forceps

Forceps are used to guide a baby through the birth canal; these metal instruments look a little like two big spoons hooked together. Often forceps are used if a baby seems to be in distress. During the pushing stage of labor, forceps can help an exhausted mother.

Vacuum Extraction

A plastic or metal suction cup is placed on the baby's head during delivery; vacuum extraction also helps speed up a delivery.

Oxytocin

Also called pitocin, it is a drug that causes contractions. It can be used to induce labor if a woman needs early delivery or has passed beyond 42 weeks of pregnancy and labor has not begun. Oxytocin also can be used to make the contractions stronger if the labor is not progressing well or the contractions are too weak. It is given intravenously to the mother a little bit at a time.

Cesarean Delivery

In a cesarean birth the baby is delivered through an incision in the mother's abdomen. Sometimes cesarean deliveries are arranged and scheduled in advance. On other occasions, the decision for a cesarean delivery will be done on an emergency basis because labor is not proceeding normally or the baby is having difficulty. Some of the reasons for cesarean delivery include:

- Cephalopelvic disproportion, in which the baby is too large to pass safely through the mother's pelvis.

- Fetal distress caused by the baby having difficulty withstanding labor or compression of the umbilical cord.

- Placental problems.

- Abnormal presentation, in which the baby lies bottom or feet first in the mother's birth canal (sometimes, the baby can be repositioned to allow a vaginal delivery).

Because cesarean deliveries are surgical procedures, recovery takes longer. Today, most clinicians encourage women who had a previous cesarean delivery to try a vaginal delivery, provided there are no reasons not to do so.

AFTER THE BABY IS BORN

Having a baby is hard work. New mothers need sleep, nourishment, quiet unpressured time to see and touch their new babies, and lots of support. The mother's body undergoes dramatic physical changes as it tries to shift gears and go back to its previous state. Many hospitals now send mothers home within the first 24 hours, which can be both a blessing and curse. While it can be comforting to be home, taking care of an infant is a 24-hour-a-day, seven-day-a-week proposition. Someone should be there to help with the beginning stages of motherhood. The body undergoes various physical changes over the next 6 weeks to return to a nonpregnant state.

Weight

Most women lose at least 13 pounds immediately after birth and an additional 3–4 pounds in the first days of the baby's life. Weight loss during the first six weeks after birth (postpartum) can be dramatic, especially for breast-feeding mothers.

Breast-feeding

Women who breast-feed need extra vitamins, minerals, and calories to support the baby. Breast milk is the best source of nutrition for a newborn baby because it has special nutrients that help the baby grow and combat diseases (see Part III, Breast-feeding). If it is not possible to breast-feed at all times, consider storing your breast milk so it can be given to the baby with a bottle.

Cramps

As the uterus contracts to its prepregnant size, cramping sensations, called afterpains, may occur in the lower abdomen for a few days. This happens more often if a woman is breast-feeding. The cramps can be relieved with a mild painkiller. However, most painkillers are passed along into breast milk and may be hazardous to the newborn. Check with your pediatrician before taking medication.

Painful Urination

After childbirth, the bladder, bowel, and pelvic floor may be tender and sore, making every trip to the bathroom something to dread. What's more, eliminating all the built up extra fluid causes more frequent urination. A warm shower can relax the muscles and help ease urination, especially with an episiotomy.

Bleeding

Vaginal bleeding occurs for several weeks; anywhere from two to six is considered normal. If the mother is breast-feeding, bleeding might stop sooner. The flow is bright red and heavy at first, turning brownish as the days pass and healing begins. Nothing should be placed in the vagina, including tampons, until healing is complete. Intercourse should be avoided.

Bowel Movements

It may take a day or so for stool to pass after delivery. Drinking lots of water, walking, and eating high fiber foods can stimulate the system and get it back in working order. Straining should be avoided. A laxative or stool softener may help.

Episiotomy
Stitches take up to 2 weeks to heal and dissolve. Soreness can be relieved by applying ice to the area and lying down to keep pressure at a minimum. The area should be kept as clean as possible.

Sexuality
A woman can resume sexual activity as soon as she has healed. The physical effects of increased levels of hormones in breast-feeding women may reduce sexual desire and function. Many women need extra lubrication. A woman may not have menstrual periods if she is breast-feeding but she could become pregnant. Select a method of birth control and begin using it soon after birth.

Postpartum Depression
About 30–80 percent of women feel down or depressed following delivery. This is called postpartum blues. These symptoms usually go away spontaneously within 10 weeks of birth, without professional help. If symptoms persist beyond that point, or if a woman thinks about hurting herself or others, she should seek professional help and possibly antidepressant medication.

Postpartum depression occurs in approximately 10 percent of women after birth. If a woman has had a previous postpartum depression, the risk increases to approximately 30 percent. Panic disorder and obsessive-compulsive disorder also may arise during the postpartum period. Some of the symptoms of postpartum depression are feelings of worthlessness, anxiety, low self-esteem, insomnia, unusual weight loss, digestive problems, social isolation, feelings of inadequacy as a mother, obsessions about the baby's health or a dissatisfying relationship, mourning the loss of her former appearance or lifestyle, and, at times, suicidal thoughts. It is important to contact your clinician for help.

Postpartum psychosis is the most severe form of postpartum psychiatric illness. It affects a very small percentage of women who deliver. Postpartum psychosis is a medical emergency and requires prompt professional attention. There may be severe agitation, insomnia, and paranoia, as well as delusions and hallucinations that can lead to suicide or an impulse to kill the baby. Despite its severity, the prognosis for full recovery from postpartum psychosis is excellent.

Resources

Every new mother should pick up at least one good book on child care. Your doctor or midwife can give recommendations.

- *The Good Housekeeping Illustrated Book of Pregnancy and Baby Care* (Hearst Books), edited by Maryann Bucknum Brinley.

- *Dr. Spock's Baby and Child Care* (Dutton) A practical, easy-to-read guide, Benjamin Spock's book has been updated at various times during the last 50 years.

- *Your Baby and Child: From Birth to Age Five* (Knopf) by Penelope Leach, a British psychologist.

- *What To Expect When You Are Expecting* (Workman) by Arlene Eisenberg, Heidi Eisenberg Murkoff, and Sandee Eisenberg Hathaway. Now part of a series of three books by this mother-daughters team, these books are packed with pertinent advice and information.

- *Caring for Your Baby and Young Child, Birth to Age 5, The Complete and Authoritative Guide* from The American Academy of Pediatrics, edited by Steven P. Shelov, M.D., F.A.A.P.

PART III

Breast-Feeding

Ruth A. Lawrence, M.D., F.A.A.P.

All mothers need to make an informed decision about how they want to feed their infant. You may have thought about it before becoming pregnant, but once the pregnancy is well established, it's important to discuss the question with your physician, your spouse, and other members of your family. If no one in your family has breast-fed before, you may find it helpful to contact one of the local groups such as International Childbirth Education Association (ICEA), La Leche League International (LLLI), or Nursing Mother's Counsel. Your obstetrician's office also can provide information about available childbirth classes in which the topic is thoroughly covered.

WHY BREAST-FEED?

The advantages of breast-feeding are numerous. Mother's milk is the ideal nutrition for a growing infant. The newborn human, one of the least mature of all the mammals, experiences the greatest brain growth in the first year of life. Human milk has the perfect ingredients to develop the brain. It has exactly the right elements to build strong bodies and to develop the brain and nervous system.

Mother's milk contains many active enzymes that help the infant to digest milk and help the infant's intestinal tract to mature and absorb the nutrients. Mother's milk, however, is more than just good nutrition. It contains antibodies to protect against infection. Breast-fed infants have fewer diarrhea and gastrointestinal infections, fewer otitis media (ear infections) and upper respiratory infections, and even have fewer urinary tract infections. They have fewer hospitalizations and fewer visits to a physician's office for illness. Infants are never allergic to their mother's milk, so breast-fed infants have fewer allergies.

Studies of chronic illness in childhood also indicate that infants who have been exclusively breast-fed for 4 or more months have less incidence of childhood onset diabetes, Crohn's disease, and childhood cancers (especially leukemia and lymphoma). In some studies, premature infants who receive their mother's milk early in life have been shown to score better on intelligence tests than those receiving only formula.

There are benefits for the mother as well. Women who breast-feed seem to have a lower incidence of breast cancer and ovarian cancer. Breast-feeders are less likely to become obese and less likely to develop calcium problems in later life than those who did not breast-feed or did not bear children.

Finally, breast-feeding can create a special relationship between mother and infant, which provides nurturing as well as nutrition and results in intimate contact many times a day.

An Informed Decision: Breast-Feeding Versus Formula

The alternative to breast-feeding is formula feeding. Today, commercially available formulas provide adequate nutrition as determined in laboratories. Most formulas (except the hypoallergenic ones) are made with cow's milk, which is altered to make it digestible for a human infant. While breast milk is always readily available at the correct concentration and temperature, formula requires preparation and the sterilization of bottles and nipples.

Some women prefer formula feeding, because their babies can be fed by other caregivers. In some ways, formula feeding is easier, because others can take over when the mother cannot be present. This may be important if the mother plans to return to school or work. Breast milk can be expressed, or pumped, from the breast and fed to the infant in a bottle or small cup.

The Role of the Father

When the infant is breast-fed, the role of the father is very important but different from the mother's. The father provides cuddling and comforting when the infant does not need to be fed. Most infants have a fussy period each day, usually in the evening (5:00 to 10:00 P.M.), when they need to be held, rocked, and stroked. The infant will nuzzle and root to be fed and may remain unsettled if she or he can smell milk. Babies settle down quickly if held by someone who is not lactating (making milk).

PRENATAL PREPARATION TO BREAST-FEEDING

As soon as pregnancy begins, the hormones produced to support the pregnancy, the placenta, and the uterus also have an effect on the breasts. The breasts begin to enlarge, the ducts that will carry the milk develop, and the cells that will produce the milk increase in number. By 16 weeks of pregnancy, the breast is ready to provide milk when the baby is born even if the infant arrives prematurely. The woman's nipples and areolas are also prepared for lactation. They become more pigmented and the Montgomery glands, which are invisible when not pregnant or lactating, enlarge and secrete a special sebaceous material that softens and lubricates the surface of the nipple and areola to protect them when the infant suckles. The nipple and areola also develop elastic tissue that will help the infant in drawing these tissues into the mouth during suckling.

If you're thinking of breast-feeding your unborn child, simply bathe and dry your breasts as you normally do. Do not use any ointments, oils, or medicines unless prescribed by your doctor. Normally, you do not need to do nipple exercises, nipple rolling, or buffing with rough cloth. These practices may cause irritation or, toward the end of pregnancy, may stimulate the uterus to contract. You should, however, have your breasts examined by an obstetrician.

Breast Examination

Breast examination is part of prenatal care. You may have questions about your breasts that you should discuss with your obstetrician early in pregnancy. Breasts, for example, come in many different sizes and shapes. Usually one is slightly bigger than the other, but a major discrepancy in size and shape should be discussed with your physician.

Of more common concern is the size and shape of the nipples, which also vary among women. If your nipples do not protrude, a simple procedure will identify their ability to become erect so they can be easily grasped by the infant and drawn into her or his mouth. Support your breast with your fingers at the level of the areola, with the thumb above. Compress the areola. Does your nipple protrude? If your nipple becomes more inverted or indented, this suggests a true inverted nipple. Discuss this with your obstetrician, who may wish to suggest some treatment after evaluating your nipples. (Some doctors prefer to wait until after delivery and rely on the infant and an electric breast pump to draw the nipple out.)

If the uterus has been very irritable or there is concern about premature delivery, it is best to delay treatment with breast shells until delivery. A *breast shell* is a simple device that consists of a plastic disc about the size of the areola that has a hole in the center for the nipple. A dome of plastic with air holes in it fits over the disc. The shell, worn under your brassiere, gently encourages the nipple to protrude. (See Figure 3.1)

Flat nipples may also be of concern. They respond to simple treatment with breast shells or an electric pump used just before the infant begins to feed. After the infant has been successfully nursing for a few days, these special procedures should no longer be necessary, as the nipple will become erect on stimulation.

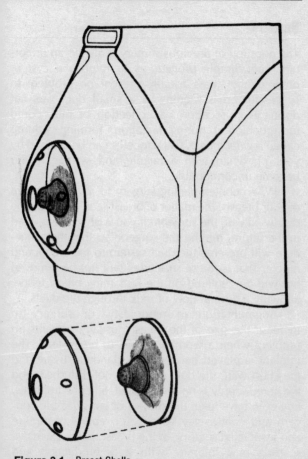

Figure 3.1   Breast Shells
Breast shells, worn under a bra, are used to encourage inverted
nipples to protrude in preparation for breast-feeding. A disk with a
hole in the center is placed over the nipple, and a small plastic
dome with air holes fits over the disk.

Surgery

The question of previous surgery is always an important one. Simple procedures to remove a cyst or other benign mass usually present no problem to successful breast-feeding. If a small duct was cut during the procedure, a collection of milk could form behind it during lactation, forming a lump called a *galactocele*. Galactoceles can be drained by your physician with a needle and syringe if you become uncomfortable.

When contemplating surgery to reduce the size of your breasts, the matter of breast-feeding should be discussed with the surgeon. If you wish to breast-feed in the future, remind the surgeon so that the procedure will preserve the duct system to the areola and nipple. That is, these structures will not be removed but will be centered on the remaining breast tissue, allowing a normal flow of milk through the ducts.

Augmentation mammoplasty, or surgery to increase the size of the breasts, usually presents no problem when a woman wishes to breast-feed. The implant is placed between the glandular tissue and the chest wall; the duct system is not disturbed, and the nerve supply is not interrupted. Silicone implants, however, have been the subject of considerable concern and controversy because of reports of rupture and associated scarring of the breast tissue. Extensive scarring may interfere with milk production and release. Whether the silicone itself is the problem remains an open question. If the implant is intact, breast-feeding is safe. If there is any question, the milk can be examined in the laboratory for the presence of silicone.

Burns to the chest wall and other causes of breast

scarring should be evaluated by your obstetrician. Breast-feeding is usually successful, and most women will find that with a little extra instruction, they can enjoy this special relationship with their infant. Your physician may refer you to another member of the staff experienced in breast-feeding or to an independent licensed lactation consultant.

Supporting the Breasts

Ordinarily, during pregnancy and lactation most women find that wearing a suitable brassiere relieves the "weighty" feeling in their breasts. Nursing bras, specially designed to allow you to feed the infant without getting completely undressed, can be purchased during the last trimester. They have adjustable shoulder straps and a long series of hooks in the back so they accommodate any changes in size that occur from the end of pregnancy into lactation. Many women wear their nursing bras day and night for weeks or even months. Avoid nursing brassieres that have narrow shoulder straps or built-in plastic-lined guards in the cup.

When lactating, it is wise to wear a disposable pad inside your bra so that milk does not leak through onto your clothing. It is also smart to avoid wearing pure silk or any other fabric that may show a ring of wetness. Many styles of blouses and dresses open in the front, have hidden zippers, or can be pulled up from the waist so that your infant can be nursed at any time or any place without undue exposure or disruption of your clothing. Flowered or print blouses have the obvious advantage of obscuring any signs of moisture.

Preparatory Classes

Infants are born knowing how to breast-feed, but women must learn; it is not a reflex. In some mammalian species, females learn by observing other breast-feeding females that live with them. Today, women in the United States may have to learn how to breast-feed from a special organization. Furthermore, their own mothers may not have any advice, because they themselves did not breast-feed. La Leche League International and the International Childbirth Education Association have local branches that can be contacted about prenatal classes and assistance after delivery.

AFTER THE BIRTH: BREAST-FEEDING IN THE FIRST FEW DAYS

Breast-feeding begins shortly after birth. Infants are born with the right reflexes and instincts to breast-feed. In a normal delivery of a healthy child, the newly born infant will find his or her way to the breast and latch on, if left undisturbed on the mother's abdomen after the umbilical cord is clamped and cut. When in the uterus, infants suck and swallow amniotic fluid during the second and third trimesters. They are born with a rooting reflex, which means they will try to suck any object that stimulates the surface around their mouths. Their sucking motion, or undulating motion of the tongue, triggers the back of the throat to swallow.

Unless you have witnessed other women breast-feeding, you may need help in properly holding your baby for feeding. Hold your infant so that she or he is facing your breasts. Rest your infant's head in the crook of your elbow and support her or his buttocks. You may want to swaddle your child in a light blanket, because it has a calming effect. Draw the infant to your breast with her or his face squarely facing it. (See Fig. 3.2) With your other hand, support your

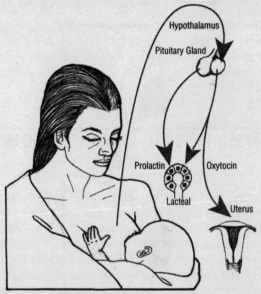

Figure 3.2   Breast-feeding
The breast-feeding cycle stimulates the production of milk in response to the infant's suckling, After delivery, a sudden drop in the hormones estrogen and progesterone begins to trigger milk production. The baby's suckling stimulates the hypothalamus and pituitary gland to release the hormones prolactin and oxytocin. These hormones in turn stimulate the production of milk and its transport through the alveoli and milk ducts. At the same time, the uterus is stimulated to contract and to begin to return to its normal size under the influence of oxytocin.

breast and compress the areola so that the infant can draw the nipple and areola into her or his mouth. (See Fig. 3.3) As the nipple and areola elongate to form a teat, the infant's tongue compresses it against the hard palate and suckles. The undulating motion of the tongue causes the milk to move along the ducts and be ejected from the nipple. (See Fig. 3.4)

You may feel comfortable supporting the breast

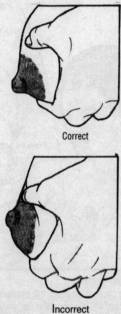

Correct

Incorrect

Figure 3.3 Positioning
To allow your baby to draw the nipple into her or his mouth, place your hand around one of your breasts with four fingers beneath the areola and your thumb on top. Gently press with fingers under the breast (top) to cause the nipple to protrude. Do not press in with your thumb (bottom), as this will tend to draw the nipple up and away from the baby's mouth.

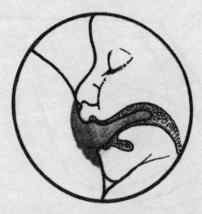

Figure 3.4 Suckling
When the baby latches onto the breast, the nipple is elongated and drawn back into her or his mouth. The baby's suckling motions stimulate the flow of milk through the milk ducts and out of the nipple toward the back of the baby's throat.

with three fingers below the breast and the thumb and index finger above and well behind the areola. (See Fig. 3.5) An alternative position is to place all four fingers below the breast and the thumb above. (See Fig. 3.6) Choose the grasp most comfortable for you, ensuring that your fingers do not block the infant from getting most of the areola in the mouth. Whether you lie down or sit up to nurse, the same principles apply: The infant's total body faces your breast, and your hand supports the breast and compresses the areola without obstructing the infant from getting a proper grasp.

To encourage the infant to latch on, stimulate the center of the infant's lower lip. (See Fig. 3.7) The rooting reflex will stimulate the infant to move forward, extend the tongue, and draw the nipple and areola

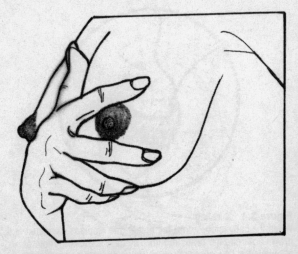

Figure 3.5 Scissors Grasp
One way to support the breast during breast-feeding is with the thumb and forefinger above the areola and the other three fingers beneath it. This is sometimes called the "scissors grasp."

into the mouth and begin suckling. If a good comfortable latch on is not achieved the first time, break the suction by slipping your finger into the corner of the infant's mouth and then repeat the process of positioning, stimulating the rooting reflex, and latching on.

The Let-Down Reflex

The infant will begin to suckle as soon as he or she is latched on. When the nipple is stimulated by the infant suckling or by a breast pump, this stimulation triggers what is known as the *let-down reflex*. The let-

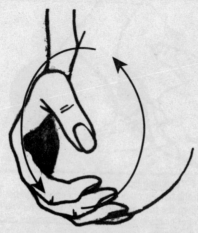

Figure 3.6 Alternate Grasp
Some women prefer to hold the breast with four fingers under-
neath the areola and the thumb on top. Choose the position that is
most comfortable and effective for you.

down reflex sends a message through the nerves in
the nipple to the mother's brain. The mother's pituitary gland releases two hormones: prolactin and
oxytocin. Prolactin stimulates the milk-producing
cells in the breast to make milk, and oxytocin stimulates the duct system to move the milk to the nipple
and eject, or let it down. (See Fig. 3.2) A little oxytocin is released when a woman hears or sees her
baby, thus a little milk will drip. A new supply of
milk, however, is not produced unless the nipple is
stimulated by the infant or a pump.

It is important in the early days of breast-feeding
to lie down or sit comfortably and to relax before
feeding the infant. Feed your baby when he or she is

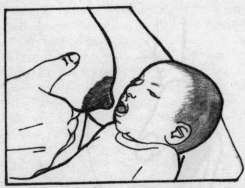

Figure 3.7 Latching On
Stimulating the baby's lower lip will help encourage her or him to latch on. When the baby is ready to feed, she or he will move forward, open her or his mouth and extend the tongue, and draw the nipple into the mouth.

ready, not when he or she has begun to cry frantically. Stress and discomfort can interfere with letting down.

You can prevent the development of sore nipples by proper positioning. If your nipples do get sore, evaluate and adjust your position. While there are several ways to hold an infant while feeding, find one or two that are best for you and your baby.

In the hospital, the nursing staff in the birthing center, postpartum floor, or newborn nursery can assist in getting you started. If you have problems such as flat or inverted nipples, a sleepy baby, or a baby with a cleft palate, talk to your physician. She or he can evaluate the situation and, if necessary, call for an appropriate consultant.

Because there are many things to learn about a

new baby, it's difficult for a new mother to retain all the information that the health care staff provides. In addition, women are often discharged from the hospital with their new babies 24 to 48 hours after birth. There is simply not enough time for the doctors and nurses to assess the newborn and its needs completely. It is important, then, to make an appointment with the baby's doctor in the 1st week after birth. Ideally, try to schedule a home visit from an office nurse practitioner or a visiting nurse who is skilled at looking at mothers and babies in the first few days postpartum.

When the Milk Comes In

At about 16 weeks of pregnancy, a small amount of milk can be expressed or may seep from the nipples. This early milk is called *colostrum*. Colostrum increases in volume so that at birth, after the placenta has been passed, the infant can suckle and obtain up to 0.5 ounce. Colostrum is yellowish, a little thicker than milk, and contains a lot of protective antibodies and cells that will protect the infant against infections and disease. It has more protein but a little less fat than later milk. Colostrum persists for 4 or 5 days and is gradually replaced by mature milk. (See Fig. 3.8) (The interim milk is called transitional milk.) Mature milk is available after about 10 days.

Right after delivery, the breasts feel soft, but over the next day, the body increases the blood supply to the breasts and they become full. As the infant nurses and receives the colostrum, the breast makes more and more fluid. About the third or fourth day after birth, you will be aware of an increase in the size of your breasts and the increased flow and change in texture and color that indicate transitional milk. This means your milk has "come in." Mothers who have nursed other infants will find that their milk comes in earlier. While some swelling and engorgement of the breast is to be expected, excessive swelling can be uncomfortable. Your physician or nurse can suggest some means of relief.

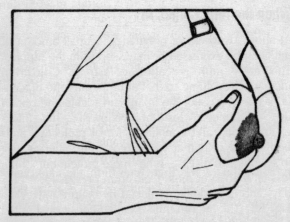

Figure 3.8 Colostrum
Colostrum is a thin, yellowish fluid that begins to be produced in the middle of pregnancy. Expressing milk can be done with the same grasp used to feed the infant.

Is Your Baby Getting Enough?

While it is not possible to measure the exact amount of milk that the infant gets at each breast-feeding, there are ways to tell if it is enough.

Feeding patterns vary, but a baby should be fed at least every 3 to 4 hours or a minimum of 6 times a day in the 1st month of life. Most breast-fed infants feed every 2 to 3 hours, resulting in 8 to 12 feedings a day. Often the infant will feed frequently for a few hours, especially between 5:00 and 10:00 P.M. and then stretch it out to 2 or 4 feedings overnight until 6:00 A.M. Feedings usually last 20 to 30 minutes, but may be shorter. The actually vigorous suckling time usually adds up to about 90 minutes a day.

Breast-fed infants should wet at least six diapers a day, soaking at least one. (It is easier to keep track of wettings with cloth diapers than with disposable ones, especially the super-absorbent kind.) The urine should be pale in color. It should not be dark, concentrated, or leave a dusty deposit. A breast-fed infant also has a bowel movement every day in the first 4 to 6 weeks. Most breast-fed infants pass a stool with every feeding, because of the physiologic stimulus to the intestinal track. Right after birth, the infant passes a substance called *meconium*, which is a dark green, almost black material that is smooth and sticky. It should be totally passed by 3 days, and stools then become green brown (transitional stools) and then yellow and seedy. Yellow, loose, and seedy is the normal breast-fed stool, and it should begin by the third or fourth day. Failure to stool every day and to have loose yellow stools by the fourth day should be reported to your pediatrician.

Failure to wet enough diapers and failure to feed long enough should also be discussed with the doctor.

Home scales are not very accurate, so take your infant to the physician's office for a weight check. Most infants lose weight after birth. A loss of 5 percent of birth weight is acceptable (5 ounces for a 7-pound baby). If the infant loses 7 to 8 percent of his or her birth weight, have the infant checked by the baby's physician. A loss of 10 percent is the maximum before aggressive interventions are introduced. Usually problems can be solved by adjusting the pattern of feeding, the frequency, or the positioning. The physician will want to check the infant every day or two until the milk supply is well established and weight gain persists. By 14 days, the infant should have returned to birth weight.

There are many community resources for nursing mothers to call for reassurance and guidance in the art of breast-feeding. La Leche League and Nursing Mother's Council have members who have nursed and who are willing to share their experiences. Management advice, however, should come from a certified licensed practitioner that your physician recommends and who will work with your physician to solve the problem.

DAY-TO-DAY BREAST-FEEDING: SPECIAL CARE AND TREATMENT

Ordinarily, no special treatment is necessary for the nipples, areola, or breasts. During normal showering or bathing, avoid putting soap directly on the nipples. Dry breasts gently but thoroughly. Between feedings, allow the milk to air dry on the skin. Bras should be kept dry and a dry nursing pad placed in the cup. As time goes on, there will be less leaking and less full-ness. This does not mean the milk has dried up but that the breast is adapting to the process of producing and releasing milk on a continual basis.

If the nipples become sore, seek help before there are cracks and further trauma. Remember, it should not hurt to breast-feed. If it does, get advice from the nursing staff or from a lactation consultant referred by your doctor.

Occasionally, a lump may appear in the breast that does not go away. (The lactating breast feels lumpy but usually the lumps change.) The lump may be a milk-filled cyst caused by a plugged duct. Gentle but firm massage will usually drain it, especially after applying warm compresses. If you become feverish or feel sick or if the lump is painful, red, and warm, it may be mastitis. Mastitis must be treated. Call your physician promptly. You may have to take special antibiotics for 10 days to 2 weeks. Continue to breast-feed on both sides; start with the unaffected side and end up fully emptying the involved side. The most important part of the treatment is *rest*. Mastitis usual-ly occurs when you have taken on too much activity or have become exhausted from caring for your baby. You'll need help with the baby and you will need to be relieved of other chores until you are rested and feel better. Hot or cold compresses will relieve local discomfort. Aspirin or ibuprofen can be taken for the fever, pain, and headache.

When the nipples become raw and painful, local treatment may be necessary. Treatment differs in different parts of the country. If the climate is very dry, as in desert areas, then treatment with bland ointments (Vitamins A and D or purified lanolin) will provide relief. In areas with high humidity, drying may help. Air drying or gentle blowing with a hair dryer on low heat and low air may be soothing. Your local health care provider will recommend the best skin treatment for the environment in which you live.

WORKING AND BREAST-FEEDING

You may have to return to work, but it is still possible to continue to breast-feed. The baby's schedule can be adjusted to fit the requirements of the job. Breast- feeding can also be adjusted, depending on your work hours, breaks, and lunch hours. Some women continue to nurse or pump so the baby receives only mother's milk. Others may provide formula and breast-feed only while at home. There are no hard-and-fast rules. The feeding should be comfortable for you, the baby, and the child care provider. For best results, you need to find safe child care where breast-feeding is understood and supported. You should be able to nurse at day care when you drop off your infant, before you leave, and when you return to pick up the child. If your job permits, you should be able to breast-feed at other times during the day. Any amount of mother's milk continues to provide special nourishment, antibodies, and protection against disease.

EDITORS AND CONTRIBUTORS

MEDICAL CO-EDITORS

ROSELYN PAYNE EPPS, M.D., M.P.H., M.A., F.A.A.P., is an expert at the National Institutes of Health, Bethesda, Maryland, and a Professor at Howard University College of Medicine, Washington, D.C. She is recognized nationally and internationally in areas of health policy and research, health promotion and disease prevention, and medical education and health service delivery. As a pioneer and leader in numerous professional and community organizations, she served, in 1991, as the first African American president of AMWA and the founding president of the AMWA Foundation.

SUSAN COBB STEWART, M.D., F.A.C.P., is an internist and gastroenterologist, and is presently Associate Medical Director at J. P. Morgan in New York, where she delivers general medical care, specialty consultations, and preventive services. She is Clinical Assistant Professor of Medicine at SUNY, Brooklyn. Since serving as President of AMWA in 1990, Dr. Stewart has continued to help AMWA shape and focus its mission in the area of women's health.

CONTRIBUTORS

Susan Aucott Ballagh, M.D., has advanced training in reproductive endocrinology and is Director of the Stanford Women's Group, Stanford Health Services. She is an Assistant Professor of Obstetrics and Gynecology at Stanford University School of Medicine, Palo Alto, California.

Barbara Bartlik, M.D., is a psychiatrist in private practice in New York City and is on staff at the Human Sexuality Teaching Program at New York Hospital-Cornell Medical Center. She has expertise in the psychiatric aspects of disorders related to the female reproductive system.

Jean L. Fourcroy, M.D., Ph.D., is a urologist with a primary interest in male reproductive endocrinology and toxicology. She is medical officer in the Division of Endocrinology and Metabolic Drug Products of the Food and Drug Administration. She is also an Assistant Professor of Surgery at the University of Health Sciences—F. Edward Hebert School of Medicine and the founder of Women in Urology. Dr. Fourcroy will serve as AMWA President in 1996.

Ruth A. Lawrence, M.D., F.A.A.P., is a Professor of Pediatrics and Professor of Obstetrics and Gynecology at the University of Rochester. A national and international authority on lactation, she is a Consultant to the Breastfeeding Advisory Group of the State of New York Department of Health and to the International Childbirth Education Association.

Katherine A. O'Hanlan, M.D., F.A.C.O.G., F.A.C.S., is an Assistant Professor of Gynecology and Obstetrics at Stanford University School of Medicine in California and Associate Director of the Gynecological Cancer Service at Stanford Medical Center.

Index